The New Generation Breast Cancer Book

The New Generation Breast Cancer Book

How to Navigate Your Diagnosis and Treatment Options—and Remain Optimistic—in an Age of Information Overload

Elisa Port, MD, FACS

Chief of Breast Surgery at The Mount Sinai Hospital
and Co-director of the Dubin Breast Center

BALLANTINE BOOKS
NEW YORK

No book can replace the diagnostic expertise and medical advice of a trusted physician. Please be certain to consult with your doctor before making any decisions that affect your health, and throughout the course of any treatment.

As of press time, the URLs displayed in this book link or refer to existing websites on the Internet. Penguin Random House LLC is not responsible for, and should not be deemed to endorse or recommend, any website other than its own or any content available on the Internet (including without limitation at any website, blog page, information page) that is not created by Penguin Random House.

A Ballantine Books Trade Paperback Original

Published in the United States by Ballantine Books, an imprint of Random House, a division of Penguin Random House LLC, New York.

BALLANTINE and the HOUSE colophon are registered trademarks of Penguin Random House LLC.

ISBN 978-1-101-88315-0
eBook ISBN 978-1-101-88314-3

Printed in the United States of America on acid-free paper

randomhousebooks.com

9 8 7 6 5 4 3 2 1

Book design by Caroline Cunningham

To my family: Jeff, "I couldn't have done any of this without you" doesn't even begin to describe my gratitude for your love and support in all things. And Zack and Lauren, you have understood from the beginning that when I am at work and not able to be with you, I am taking care of other mommies so that they can go home to their families. I love you dearly.

To my parents: Jeff and Loni Rush, for your love and support from the beginning, I will be forever grateful.

To Eva and Glenn Dubin: You are my partners in the Dubin Breast Center, and together we created a model for what breast cancer care can and should be.

And to my patients: you inspired me to write this book, continue to inspire me every day, and have given me the honor of taking care of you.

Contents

Introduction

The last feeling you have when you're told that you—or someone you love—has breast cancer? Lucky.

And though it feels like it's so common—one in three of *all* new cancer cases diagnosed each year in women is a breast cancer—the notion that you'll have lots of company offers little comfort.

But here's the reality: if you have been diagnosed with breast cancer, you have every reason to be optimistic. At no point in history has the survival rate from breast cancer been better: overall survival from breast cancer now approaches 90 percent. Which means that if you're diagnosed with breast cancer, chances are you will survive and thrive. Even more heartening is that over the last decade the death rate from breast cancer has dropped significantly each year, and that trend continues strongly.

Perhaps you've heard that, thanks to mammograms and early detection, if you are diagnosed with breast cancer today, it will most likely be early stage, which is extremely treatable and curable. And you may know that even for women diagnosed at more advanced stages, there are a growing number of cutting-edge treatment options available, with more on the way each year. But what you may not have heard is that for everyone, we are using less invasive surgery and treatments while still achieving better outcomes, and offering more options for reconstruction than ever before.

All this is the good news. The bad news is that it can be hard for women to hear this message of optimism against all the background noise.

At forty-eight, Katherine* was leading a have-it-all kind of life that, as far as she was concerned, couldn't get much fuller. She held a demanding job in human relations for a large tech company; her husband worked full-time, and like Katherine's, his job involved lots of travel. Her two girls, ages thirteen and fifteen, were just hitting all the emotional potholes that come with being teenagers. Her seventy-six-year-old mother, who lived five hundred miles away, had recently had heart valve replacement surgery, and Katherine had spent the last few weeks figuring out how to find her good nursing care.

She was juggling it all at a hundred miles an hour, like so many of us do. Then, in a single moment, the daily rhythm of life faded into the background. After her yearly routine mammogram, she was told there was an "abnormality" and that she had to have a biopsy. When the biopsy results came back, I had to tell Katherine the four words that no woman wants to hear: "You have breast cancer."

Katherine responded to the news as so many women that I see do, and perhaps as you have as well. After the initial shock, she, her husband, and I huddled together in my office and spent a long time discussing her options and making some important decisions. By the end of it, Katherine was drained, for sure, but relieved to have a clear plan of action. She felt reassured by the process and comfortable in her treatment plan, and she could turn her focus and her energies to her family and the upcoming surgery. She left my office confident that she would be okay and optimistic about her future.

But within a day or two of our visit, something happened that upset Katherine's clarity and balance. I completely understood what was going on—I see this in my office all the time.

What happened was this: after she left my office, Katherine headed

---

* The case examples in this book are compilations of patient and case details that I have seen and treated. The medical information is accurate; the names and identifying characteristics are changed in order to disguise the patients.

home and started Googling just about everything having to do with her diagnosis, and she began second-guessing everything. Two days after our meeting, she called me apologetically saying she had a long list of questions she hadn't known to ask during our first meeting, and could she come to see me again? Fortunately, I was able to see her the next day. The Katherine who walked in was a different person. She had a three-inch stack of computer printouts highlighted in three different colors, with Post-it notes flapping off particular pages. Her eyes were bloodshot, and she looked like she hadn't slept since I saw her last. She seemed utterly perplexed and defeated.

And then she began. She'd heard there was a new drug that could be given before surgery to reduce the size of the cancer; what did I think of that? (The drug wasn't right for her kind of cancer.) She had been to a really well-respected website where all the women on it said mastectomy would give her a better survival rate than lumpectomy. (Absolutely not true. In Katherine's case, the odds were the same.) She had read that it was a good idea to have her other breast removed too so she would have the lowest likelihood of recurrence. (Again, not at all true in her case.)

I wasn't surprised by Katherine's questions. Not only have a woman's odds of surviving and living a full and long life after a breast cancer diagnosis increased, but so have the number of sources for obtaining information. Well-meaning friends send emails linking you to websites with a note in the subject line that says "Must Read." Family members pass along "required" reading, or insist that they introduce you to their old friend who has a doctor you must see or a survival story you must hear. And while having a disease that is so common—affecting one in eight women—can be an advantage because so much is known about it, it can also be a problem: *everyone* knows something about breast cancer, knows someone you should call, or knows someone who knows someone.

Thirty years ago, when our mothers and grandmothers were diagnosed, women didn't even talk about "the big C." Or if they did, they would literally whisper the word "cancer." Back then, the word "breast" couldn't even be used in a magazine advertisement! Twenty years ago, when I first entered the breast cancer field, access to information about breast cancer for the general public was still fairly limited. There was very little information online, only a few books on the market, and significantly fewer options for treatment.

Fast-forward to today. There is no shortage of information out there if you are newly diagnosed with breast cancer, including books like this one. But the omnipresent Internet is definitely the game changer, and not always in a good way. When you type the words "breast cancer" into your browser, you're faced with literally millions of pages. And a breast cancer diagnosis is no longer spoken of in hushed tones; it is often blogged and tweeted about by women chronicling their journey through treatment, sending selfies from the chemo chair for all to see. I applaud those women for finding high-tech ways to cope, and for their sincere efforts to help others get through it as well. But as you may already have seen, the problem isn't access to information anymore; instead, it's too much information, with no filter. Some of what you can find online is credible; some isn't. Some information will be relevant; most won't be. Most important, the critical information that you need to make decisions for *yourself and your particular case* is actually quite limited relative to the huge amount of information that's out there. Getting information should be empowering, but too much information without the correct guidance to figure out its relevance can have the opposite effect.

Katherine and I spent as much time as she needed addressing all of the issues she'd raised, and a significant amount of time revisiting her options. I commended her on her diligence—but then refocused her on what was important: her particular case. At the end of our discussion, what Katherine understood was that while doing her research was an important part of the process, all of the information she had gathered came with a catch: without the right guidance, it was a challenge to assess its relevance to her particular case. We had to make those determinations together. Our discussions continued until Katherine regained her comfort and expressed genuine confidence in the plan we had initially established just for her. I confirmed for her that the treatment options we had were very likely to give her an excellent outcome, and Katherine left my office that day knowing that the odds of cure in her case—and for most women diagnosed with breast cancer today—were overwhelmingly in her favor, and that she was on the right path toward wellness.

It's stories like Katherine's—and literally thousands of others from the patients I've had the privilege to treat over the years—that have led me to write this book. The mental high-wire act women face—empowered to seek out information 24/7, but also overwhelmed by the TMI factor—can be exhausting. There's no question that a woman diagnosed with breast cancer today faces a very different world than a woman diagnosed in decades past, and most women, I think, could use some guidance on how to navigate this world. Furthermore, many will not be able to get in to see a doctor as quickly as Katherine was able to with me. For many women newly diagnosed with breast cancer, it can be days, if not weeks, before a visit to a doctor who can provide any meaningful information to you and your family about your particular case. What I have been told by so many patients is that the time between diagnosis and actually meeting with the doctor and developing a plan of attack is the toughest. It is during this period when you (and often your spouse or family) feel so vulnerable, with no one to answer your questions. This is the time when, desperate for information, you can end up burning the midnight oil (who can sleep after receiving a diagnosis of breast cancer?) trolling the Internet for any meaningful information you might find.

And that's where this book comes in. Whether you are concerned about a lump, are worried about a friend, or have already been diagnosed with breast cancer, there is a way to travel this road knowing that you have every reason to be optimistic. My goal with my patients—and now with my readers—is to provide guidance from an insider on all aspects of breast cancer treatment and care. This is where you can go to check in and make sure you're on the right path at every step of your journey, so that you can come out on the other side with your health and positive outlook intact, leaving the background noise behind. I will help you set your priorities and pare down your list of concerns to the ones that are relevant to you and your particular situation. I hope to also arm you with a honed sense of what questions you need to ask and keep asking throughout your treatment and experience with breast cancer.

To start with, here are a few key pieces of advice and strategy. I will discuss these ideas and themes throughout this book, but to get you oriented and started on your fact gathering and decision making, these are the most important things you need to do at the outset:

1. **Find the right team.** Breast cancer care is multidisciplinary, which means that different doctors from different disciplines (surgery, medicine, radiation, plastic surgery, and others) may be involved in different aspects of your care. And just to make it potentially more complicated, the number and types of different doctors and specialists that may be involved with your care will vary from person to person and from case to case. Not *all* women need to see *all* these different types of doctors. That's why navigating your path through breast cancer can be particularly confusing and overwhelming, but with the right guidance it's not. To start, it's important to know that almost all treatment for breast cancer is sequential. For example, if it's determined that you'll need surgery, chemotherapy, and radiation, you'll get these treatments one after the other, not at the same time, and therefore will have a sequence of different doctors running the show at different points in the course of your care. Who comes first? How do you make your way from one doctor to the next? Starting in chapter 4, you will learn about the order in which you will be likely to meet and interface with the members of your treatment team—including surgeon, plastic surgeon, medical oncologist, radiologist, and others—because even at the outset, when you've just been diagnosed, you'll want to assemble a team that you feel confident and comfortable with. I'll explain how.

2. **Do everything you can to see doctors who specialize in breast cancer.** When patients are taken care of by doctors in centers that treat more cancer—known as high-volume centers—the results are better. In one study investigating breast surgery outcomes related to volume, only 7 percent of surgeons met the criteria for performing a "high volume" of breast surgery (more than fifty cases per year), and only 25 percent of patients had their surgery performed by a high-volume breast surgeon. The other 75 percent had surgery with a medium- to low-volume surgeon, many of whom performed fewer than two breast procedures per month. Here's why that matters: those patients who went to high-volume breast surgeons were significantly more likely to be offered and receive the most advanced breast surgery

options, and thus better treatment.* It makes sense: the more experience someone has regularly performing a task—whether it's a haircut, a business deal, or a particular type of surgery—the higher likelihood of a better result. This is particularly true for breast cancer care today. With all the advances that have already been made, all the different treatment options out there, and more progress occurring each year, there *is* so much to know and so much to keep current on when it comes to breast cancer (you should see the stack of medical journals and publications on my nightstand). So if at all possible, avoid doctors who "dabble" in breast cancer care as part of their practice. The doctor who dabbles, treating only a few patients per month or even per year, may not have the up-to-date knowledge base to provide the best recommendations for treatment. For most doctors, high volume is usually achieved by becoming a specialist. A specialist is someone who, after receiving general training, goes on to get additional, advanced training in one specific area, or someone who chooses to focus his or her practice on one particular disease or organ system. So breast cancer care is best provided by specialists who have chosen to focus *only* on breast cancer in all its forms and all its treatments. With each member of the team, if at all possible, it'll be key to find a specialist: someone who focuses primarily or completely on breast cancer within his or her particular field. So a breast radiologist spends most of his or her time looking at mammograms and all of the other imaging studies related to diagnosing breast cancer. A breast surgeon is a surgeon who devotes most if not all of his or her practice to performing breast surgery. Seeking out high-volume specialists is one way to stack the odds in your favor for getting the best breast cancer care.

3. **Along the way, make sure you choose doctors you feel you can work with to make decisions.** When you are diagnosed with breast cancer, you will have many choices to make: Lumpectomy or mastectomy? Chemotherapy or no chemotherapy? What

---

* McDermott AM, Wall DM, Waters PS et al. Surgeon and breast unit volume-outcome relationships in breast cancer surgery and treatment. *Annals of Surgery,* 2013.

about additional treatments? And so many more. More than with any other disease type, decision making in breast cancer care is often *both* medical *and* personal. As I frequently tell patients, "I may be the expert in cancer, but you are the expert in *you*." And because we're talking about an area of a woman's anatomy that is both extremely visible and very personal (and often an essential part of her sense of herself as woman), there's a huge amount at stake. When you get the information you need provided by the right specialists, you can feel calm and optimistic, which in turn will maximize your chances of making the best decisions, for now and for your future.

4. **Know that it's not an emergency.** It's hard *not* to imagine that cancer is growing and spreading by the minute, the hour, and the day, and most women and their families believe that when you are diagnosed with breast cancer, time is of the essence. It's important to know that this is not how cancer works. You may be surprised to learn that even a cancer that seems to have just "popped up out of nowhere" has grown over the course of months to years. With rare exceptions, a new breast cancer diagnosis is not a medical emergency, so it's okay to take a deep breath and allow yourself some time to formulate a plan. Don't feel desperate to get in to see the first doctor who will give you an appointment; it is certainly safe to wait days or weeks to get to the *right* doctors in the *right* centers.

5. **Always, always, always remember that no two cases are the same.** The only way to determine what's right for you is to arm yourself with the facts, discuss them with a doctor you trust, and then listen to *your own voice* above all. With breast cancer, every case is different. And even two women who *seem* to have the same diagnosis may have cases that differ in subtle ways that make a big difference in treatment options or recommendations. Because of this, there is a limit to what one can learn about her disease from the Internet, an article, or even a friend who seems to have "exactly the same thing." I think it is safe to say that when it comes to breast cancer, one size does not fit all—it doesn't even fit most. As one of my patients, Jane, said to me rel-

atively soon after her diagnosis, "If I hear one more person tell me what she would do if she were me, I am going to lose it! How does anyone know what they would do if they were in my situation? And even if they were in the same situation, they're not me!" So in this book, you will learn how to get the facts that pertain to you and your case, which will enable and empower you to move ahead with your care.

6. **Focus on what matters and tune out the background noise.** How do you do that when there *is* so much information out there? It's unrealistic to expect to insulate yourself completely from the onslaught of information and advice headed your way, but in this book you will learn strategies for how to maintain optimism and a positive outlook in the face of the storm. How do you do that? By learning to let some of the information roll off you, by differentiating fact from fiction, and by getting a preview of the many myths out there related to breast cancer, and understanding how to dispel them. And if you can succeed at the first, second, and third items on this list—finding the right team, making sure your doctors are specialists, and having medical providers you're comfortable with—the number of questions you need to research on your own should be reduced, *and* you will have reliable, trusted specialists in your corner to turn to with your concerns.

These strategies are important to keep in mind as you go through each phase of your care, and you will find them reiterated in the context of each chapter of the book. The early chapters are about screening, diagnosis, and prevention. From there, you'll learn about the steps you're likely to encounter if you have a breast cancer diagnosis, including an explanation of the different types of tumors and the implications for treatment. Next, I provide explanations of each of the various types of surgery that might be offered and the different options for medical and radiation treatment after surgery. In the world of breast cancer today, many patients are interested in knowing more about participation in research studies, understanding which lifestyle factors influence their diagnosis and treatment, and learning about the role of complementary or alternative medicine and even spirituality in their care and follow-up. So there are chapters addressing each of these important subjects.

Other topics, including how your diagnosis of breast cancer might impact other members of the family and their own risk, and the rare scenario of male breast cancer, are addressed in their own chapters. Even in the early phases of diagnosis and treatment, many women are already thinking ahead, past treatment, and wonder about what their follow-up care will be like, how they will be monitored, and what would happen if their cancer did come back. Further chapters will address these issues. At the end of the book you will find a glossary of the important terms you will learn from each chapter, and an appendix of FAQs for family members and friends. And although I advise patients to be wary of information found online (as it's so hard to apply to any individual case), I do offer a short list of online resources and organizations I find reliable and authoritative, all the more so when you know—from having read this book—what you are specifically looking for.

Within each chapter you will find sidebars headed "Need to Know" and "A Word to the Wise." These highlight specific points and pieces of information that will give you the edge in your care. Because this book is all about getting the facts and tuning out common misconceptions related to breast cancer (there are so many of them!), in many chapters you will find "Myths" related to that topic, along with explanations as to why they are just that—myths. And "The Takeaway," at the end of every chapter, will highlight the main points discussed so you know you have gotten a clear sense of the main messages.

Every day I walk into the lives of women newly diagnosed with breast cancer and get to know whatever I can about them in order to best guide them through what is undoubtedly one of the most intense periods of their lives. For a short period of time, I play a critical role in helping people I have just met and barely know make life-changing decisions for themselves. Again, with breast cancer there is no one plan that fits all, and of course there is no one guaranteed outcome for all. It's certainly true that some women—too many women—do not survive this potentially deadly disease, and too many breast cancer stories do not have a happy ending. But the prospects in today's world are better than ever. And more often than not, I am able to show my patients that with the right treatment and the right approach, we can all be optimistic. For patients newly diagnosed with breast cancer, we do have so much to offer: better treatments right now, with more becoming available all the time thanks to research and novel technology; better survival rates, even with less invasive surgery and treatments; and more attention to cosmetic outcomes, achieving excellent results. And there are many top-notch centers across the country that encompass all these aspects of care.

And Katherine? As I've said, she left my office that day feeling much, much better, and in the following days she focused on spending time with her family. On the day of surgery, she walked into the operating room ready and confident. Smiling at me, she said, "Let's do this."

The New
Generation Breast
Cancer Book

CHAPTER 1

What *Every* Woman Should Know

the risks we all face, the rewards we get from screening and prevention

You may be coming to this book from any one of a variety of different situations. Perhaps you are interested in learning more about breast cancer in general (after all, it is *the* most common solid tumor to affect women in the United States). Maybe you consider yourself to be at risk for the disease and are trying to arm yourself with the best information for the future, or you have a family member or friend whom you are hoping to support in her diagnosis. For the majority of readers, however, the most likely scenario is that you yourself have been diagnosed with breast cancer or have found something that has a high likelihood of turning out to be breast cancer. If that's the case, then you may think that you should just skip over this chapter. Why read about risk for breast cancer or how to detect it when you've already been found to have it? In fact, the information in this chapter is still relevant to you. Understanding the risk factors that may or may not have contributed to your diagnosis could be important. You'll also learn about mammograms and other different types of imaging that can still come into play even *after* you have received a diagnosis of breast cancer and in the years ahead.

Mammograms

For many women, the diagnosis of breast cancer starts with a mammogram. These women in particular usually do not need much convincing of the value of mammograms in the early detection of breast cancer. Over the past few years, however, there has been a huge amount of conflicting information out there regarding mammograms, leaving many other women feeling uncertain and confused. As a breast cancer surgeon and specialist, I'm often asked to speak to the general public about issues surrounding breast cancer screening, treatment, and care. Some of the most common questions I get during the Q&A portion go something like this:

> "My sister was diagnosed with breast cancer when she felt a lump one month after a normal mammogram. Why should I get one if it didn't work for her?"

> "I have a friend who was diagnosed with breast cancer at age thirty-eight, before she had even started mammograms. Shouldn't we all be starting earlier?"

> "I heard that sonograms and MRIs are better than mammograms at picking up cancers in women with dense breasts. Why aren't they recommended for all women?"

It doesn't surprise me that so many women have so many questions about mammograms and screening: they are looking for answers on some very controversial issues.

Mammograms aren't flawless—no test is. Mammograms have been associated with *both* underdiagnosis (missing cancer) and overdiagnosis (when we find things on a mammogram that, if left alone, would not have caused a problem). Hence the frequent controversy about when and whether to use them. But even when all these variables are taken into account, mammograms are still the best tool currently available for identifying breast cancer in the vast majority of women.

It's important to get the facts straight, beginning with this one: the mammogram is the *only* test that has been shown to decrease the actual risk of dying from breast cancer by detecting cancer earlier—effectively reducing mortality by 15 percent or more in women from ages forty to seventy.

And here's a lesser-known fact: 80 to 90 percent of women diagnosed with breast cancer have *no* preexisting risk factors—no family history, no genetic issue, nothing. So we are *all* at risk, and that's why appropriate screening is relevant to all women.

When we look at the breast cancer cure rate, the good news is that it has increased substantially in the past few decades. To a large degree, this is because of early detection—a direct result of better screening, primarily with mammograms. Currently over 60 percent of newly diagnosed breast cancers are early stage. These cancers are localized, and are usually detected by mammography *before* a woman or her doctor could feel anything on examination. So with all the conflicting information out there, it can be easy to lose sight of the bottom line here: mammograms help to detect breast cancer earlier and save lives.

Mammograms: what to expect

A mammogram is an X-ray of the breasts. Most often—including during a routine, annual mammogram—both breasts are X-rayed. This is called a bilateral mammogram, and two pictures are taken of each breast, resulting in a total of four pictures. A unilateral mammogram (just one side, right or left) consists of two pictures. There are a variety of different reasons why a woman may need a mammogram on only one side: occasionally a follow-up at a shorter interval, usually six months, for one side only will be needed to make sure something we saw previously is indeed normal or has not changed. In addition, for women who have had a prior breast cancer and had one breast removed, we only perform mammograms on the one remaining breast. Finally, if a recent bilateral mammogram was normal but a few months later a woman feels a lump on self-examination, repeating the mammogram just on that one side might be needed. In any case, when a mammogram is done, the breast is pressed between two paddles to flatten out the breast tissue, and the entire process of positioning and shooting the picture takes about a minute for each picture, or a couple of minutes for each side. I don't think anyone would argue that having your breast pressed between two paddles is exactly *pleasant*. Women do sometimes complain that mammograms are painful or at least uncomfortable, and there are many jokes circulating about how men could never tolerate the same procedure on certain parts of *their* anatomy. But the discomfort should be short and tolerable, especially at a mammography facility with experienced, well-trained technicians. If you are someone with especially sensitive breasts, discomfort may be minimized by making sure your mammogram is not scheduled right before or during your menstrual period, when breasts are usually most sensitive.

On a mammogram, cancers typically show up as white, irregular spots against the darker background of regular, mostly fatty breast tissue. Denser *normal* breast tissue also shows up as whiter, so in dense breasts it can be harder to see the white cancer against a white background (imagine trying to spot a polar bear in a snowstorm). If you do have dense breasts (very common in younger women), you may get a recommendation for additional tests, such as a sonogram, and you also may want to make sure that you are getting a *digital* mammogram. Digital mammograms have been shown to be better at picking up cancers in younger women with denser breast tissue. Other findings that we look for on a mammogram that could indicate cancer are areas of calcifications, which are tiny clusters of white spots, almost like grains of salt grouped together. And lastly, an area of asymmetry, where the tissue looks distorted or pulled, especially if different from what is seen in the other breast, could raise suspicion for a cancer as well.

One of the most exciting new developments currently available is 3-D mammography. Although it is associated with a slightly higher dose of radiation exposure with each mammogram, the 3-D images that we capture extend through the breast, section by section, in great detail. Looking at the results is a little like looking through the pages of a book, and we can pick up more cancers that are hidden among overlapping dense breast tissue as a result. In addition, 3-D mammograms have been shown to significantly reduce callbacks for additional tests, which means fewer scary phone calls and less nail-biting time for you. This new mammography technique has been widely integrated into many practices, but not everywhere.

**MYTH: "If you don't have a family history of breast cancer, then
    you are not really at risk and there's no reason to start
    mammograms at forty."**
The *normal* screening guidelines are for women at *average* risk for breast
cancer. The reality is that 80 to 90 percent of women diagnosed with
breast cancer have *no* special risk factors. So we are *all* at risk, and that's
why appropriate screening is relevant to all women.

Why not start screening earlier?
There are some women in a higher risk group who do need to start
screening for breast cancer earlier than forty (see below for more on
this). But for women at *average* risk, screening beginning at forty is
standard. Some doctors do order baseline mammograms for their
average-risk patients prior to age forty, usually after seeing a few upsetting cases of breast cancer diagnosed in very young women. These
exceptional cases stand out in the minds of physicians, and, not wanting to miss a cancer, ever, they sometimes order mammograms earlier
than recommended for their other patients. But seeing one thirty-five-
year-old with breast cancer does not necessarily mean that all thirty-
five-year-olds should get a mammogram earlier. Overall, for women
turning thirty, less than 1 percent would be expected to develop breast

cancer over the ensuing ten years. So again, beginning testing at forty for most women is the norm, and your risk of missing a cancer by not doing mammograms before forty is extremely low. If you are going to get a mammogram prior to age forty and don't have a family history, consider the facts I'll lay out below about the pros and cons of earlier mammography, and make sure you discuss the pros and cons with the doctor who is ordering it.

Why not start screening later?

There are many people who sincerely believe that it's okay to start mammograms later, at age fifty. And it's important to know that in some countries, such as in the UK, the current recommended age to start mammograms *is* age fifty, despite data showing a benefit for starting earlier. Part of the recent controversy over mammograms can be traced back to a recommendation made in November 2009 by the United States Preventive Services Task Force (USPSTF) to begin screening later, starting at age fifty—a change from their previous recommendation to start at forty. The USPSTF is a committee charged with reviewing data and making recommendations for health care organizations regarding the relative benefits of various services, and many women and their doctors are strongly influenced by this group's recommendations.

Here's why screening beginning at age forty remains my recommendation and the recommendation of many other physicians and breast cancer organizations around the country. Simply put, we don't accept the rationale behind the USPSTF's 2009 recommendation. The USPSTF seems to have made its new recommendation largely based on data indicating that women in their forties have a higher number of callbacks for additional pictures and biopsies after mammograms, many of which prove to be insignificant (also known as false positives). A false positive result means that a concerning finding was identified but then did not prove to be cancer—the radiology equivalent of a false alarm. The USPSTF reasoned that if we stopped doing mammograms in this group, we would be sparing a lot of women a lot of unnecessary tests and everything bad that goes with them (unnecessary biopsy in some cases, and anxiety and worry while waiting for the results). While additional tests, especially biopsies, can be stressful and even unpleasant for women, as far as I'm concerned, this isn't enough of a reason to forgo mammograms in the forty-to-fifty age group. The main reason: the proven reduction in mortality of 15 percent or more for women ages forty to fifty who have regular mammograms. That is a significant percentage, translating into tens of thousands of lives saved each year. And I'm not alone in this reasoning. The USPSTF findings from November 2009 have been dismissed and decried by almost every major medical professional society, national cancer organization, and breast cancer advocacy group in the United States.

A WORD TO THE WISE

While lives saved is the most important measure of a screening test's success, there are other potential benefits of screening with mammography that are less frequently publicized but extremely important as well. What about the fact that a cancer found by mammogram, before it is picked up by self-exam, is less likely to require extensive surgery? And less extensive surgery, such as lumpectomy, is associated with quicker recovery and minimal overall change in appearance. Plus women with smaller, earlier cancers, such as those detected by mammogram, may be less likely to require subsequent aggressive treatment, such as chemotherapy. The point is that picking up cancer earlier is better for so many reasons, and that's what mammograms do. Mammograms are worth it, even if they do sometimes lead to additional and unnecessary testing.

MYTH: "Mammograms don't reduce cancer mortality."

Occasionally I hear women say, "Mammograms prevent breast cancer." It's important to clarify: mammograms don't actually *prevent* breast cancer from developing, but they do reduce the risk of dying from breast cancer by detecting it early in the vast majority of cases. Many women have seen or heard of studies that suggest mammograms don't reduce cancer mortality. You may feel that this is enough of a reason to delay getting a yearly mammogram, or not getting one at all. After all, if it won't increase survival, why bother with the test?

Yes, it's true that there have been various studies claiming to prove that mammograms do not reduce cancer mortality in significant enough numbers to warrant mammogram recommendations as they currently stand. The most recent of these, in 2014, highlighted the findings from a study done on screening mammography conducted over thirty years ago in Canada. This one study did *not* show a survival benefit associated with regular mammograms. What much of the recent coverage of the thirty-year-old data did not mention, however, was that this trial had largely been discredited due to, among other factors, the poor quality of the mammography equipment used and problems with the randomization of the selection process (where more women with obvious cancer may have been pushed toward the mammography group). Despite these criticisms and the fact that it is the *only* study that *did not* show a survival benefit, the trial continues to make headlines, calling into question the benefit of mammograms. And again the response from those of us on the front lines of cancer treatment and cure was that one flawed trial from over thirty years ago should not change recommendations for women today.

At what age is it okay to *stop* getting mammograms?

Of all of the trials that showed that mammography reduces the risk of breast cancer mortality, very few included women over the age of seventy. Remember, most of these studies were performed in the 1970s, when the average woman was only expected to live to her early seventies! So while there is little actual data to suggest screening mammograms benefit women over seventy, this is probably because the benefits in this age group have not been adequately studied.

Today, the life span of the *average* woman is well into her eighties; more impressively, a woman who lives to be eighty-five will most likely live well into her nineties. When making decisions regarding continuing screening with mammography, it's important to take into consideration not only *chronologic* age but *physiologic* age as well. In other words, we ask ourselves: if we find something on the mammogram, is the person healthy enough to tolerate further tests and possibly surgery? If the answer is no and our patient's other significant health issues will most likely limit long-term survival, then screening with a mammogram to identify an early breast cancer is probably of very limited added benefit. Conversely, if the expectation at any age is for long-term health and good quality of life, there is no reason *not* to get a mammogram with the same goal of early detection of breast cancer. I have many patients who are very healthy and spry well into their eighties, and for these women I do recommend mammograms, knowing that there is a high likelihood of them living well into their nineties. So the decision to have a mammogram (or to stop getting them) in the older age group needs to be determined on a case-by-case basis by a woman and her doctor.

When earlier screening *is* necessary, and the factors that increase risk

It bears repeating: women at average risk for breast cancer should get their first mammogram at age forty. However, even the word "average" denotes a range. And you might have risk factors that elevate you to slightly higher than average risk. What then?

Assessing individual risk is complicated and sometimes involves mathematical modeling in order to zero in on an individual's true level of risk. The Gail model is one commonly used tool for assessing risk that you may hear about, and there are others as well, such as the Tyrer-Cuzick model and BRCA-PRO. Many are available online (see the links to online resources at the back of the book), but it would be hard to go online and figure out how to input appropriate data and use these models yourself. More important, the results and their significance may be difficult for a layperson to interpret. Most breast specialists and even many primary care doctors and gynecologists know how to use these models and discuss the results, so in general my advice is to work with a doctor when trying to figure out your personal level of risk for developing breast cancer. Many specialized breast centers have high-risk programs to evaluate women who think they may be at increased risk for breast cancer, thereby enabling physicians to make more personalized recommendations for screening and prevention.

It's worth keeping in mind that most women tend to overestimate their risk of developing breast cancer because the disease is so common and everyone knows someone who has been affected. So getting a true understanding of one's risk—average, moderately increased, high, extremely high—is critical. A trusted physician can ask you important detailed questions about your family and medical history, assess your personal risk factors, perform risk modeling, and give you a realistic sense of your personal risk for breast cancer and whether or not early or additional screening is appropriate.

NEED TO KNOW

For women with a family history of breast cancer, the general recommendation is to start getting mammograms *ten years younger than when your youngest relative was diagnosed*. So if your mother was diagnosed at age forty-seven, you might consider starting to get mammograms at age thirty-seven.

Here are the main risk factors to know about in terms of early screening:

1. **Family history.** In the majority of cases, additional risk is due to breast cancer in the family. While it's true that a family history of breast cancer *does* increase your risk of getting the disease, it's important to remember that the degree of increased risk varies. Sometimes a woman's family history gives her a minimally increased risk, and so there's no need to screen earlier. Sometimes she may have a significantly higher risk, in which case early screening is important. The factors that your doctor will take into account when recommending early screening include the number of relatives with breast cancer, the closeness of those relatives (sister or mother versus second cousin once removed), and the age at which those relatives were diagnosed. As an example, if your grandmother was diagnosed with breast cancer at age seventy-seven, the increase in your risk of breast cancer would probably be minimal. If your two sisters both developed breast cancer before age forty-five, then this would put you at substantially increased risk. Many women have a family history of breast cancer where the degree of increased risk for other family members is not so clear-cut. For example, if you have an aunt with

breast cancer at age fifty, you might understandably be totally unsure as to where this puts you in the big picture of breast cancer
risk. In these types of situations, the effect on risk can be quite
variable, and you simply have to review your family history as
well as other risk factors with a specialist to get an accurate assessment of what your particular family history means for *you*.

2. **Atypia and LCIS.** Many women who have suspicious findings on
their imaging studies or feel a lump will undergo breast biopsies.
Most of these biopsies will show normal findings. Sometimes a
biopsy will show some cell changes that, while not cancer itself,
indicate an increased risk for developing a future breast cancer.
Two types of cell changes are called atypia and LCIS. For women
who are found to have atypia, their risk of getting breast cancer
over their lifetimes is mildly elevated to approximately 15 percent. LCIS stands for lobular carcinoma in situ. Despite having a
name that includes the word "carcinoma," LCIS is *not* breast cancer and does not turn into breast cancer. But it does moderately
increase one's risk of getting a future breast cancer, to approximately 20 percent.

3. **Hormonal exposure and reproductive factors.** These can include getting your period early in life, not having children or having children later in life, late onset of menopause, not
breastfeeding, and taking certain types of hormone replacement
therapy. Most of these factors in and of themselves do not increase breast cancer risk substantially, but put some of them together and the risk can add up. For example, a forty-five-year-old
woman who first got her period at age ten and had her first child
after age thirty has an estimated lifetime risk of developing breast
cancer of approximately 15 percent, which is slightly higher than
the average woman's (approximately 10 to 12 percent).

4. **When family history is hard to assess.** What if you were adopted and have no idea of your biological family's medical history? What if there haven't been many female ancestors in your
family for generations (your mother died at a young age of other
causes and had three brothers, and your father was an only
child)? It can be hard to tell with family backgrounds such as
these whether or not someone has a family history of breast can-

cer. Your doctor can help you determine whether the lack of information regarding family history is enough to warrant further assessment.

5. **Women genetically predisposed to breast cancer as a result of harboring a BRCA-1 or BRCA-2 mutation.** There are two factors that put women at the highest risk for developing breast cancer, and one of these is having a BRCA-1 or BRCA-2 mutation. Women in this category have an 80 percent risk or higher of developing breast cancer in their lifetimes, and a 20 to 40 percent chance of developing ovarian cancer. And while the most common age to be diagnosed with breast cancer for the average woman is in her sixties or seventies, for women with BRCA mutations, the average age of diagnosis is in their forties (roughly twenty years earlier). For these women, screening should begin at approximately age twenty-five. It's important to realize that women with BRCA mutations represent only a very small group of women who get breast cancer, and even among women with a family history, most do not have these mutations. So not all women diagnosed, even those with a family history, require testing for this gene. However, if you have been diagnosed with a BRCA mutation, I definitely recommend early screening. (For additional information on BRCA mutations, see chapter 15.)

6. **Women who have received chest wall radiation in the past, especially if that radiation was received at a young age.** This is the second group at highest risk. With many cancer treatments, there is a component of robbing Peter to pay Paul. In other words, we often give treatments to cure a life-threatening cancer today knowing that there may be side effects that will increase the risk of developing another cancer down the line. Hodgkin's disease is a type of lymphoma, and its treatment can involve chemotherapy, radiation, or both. When chest wall radiation is necessary to treat Hodgkin's disease in girls and young women, especially during the critical phase of breast development in the teenage years, there is an increased risk of developing breast cancer—as much as forty times that of the average woman. A young woman treated for Hodgkin's disease in her teens should start screening for breast cancer as early as her twenties, as the devel-

opment of the breast cancer can be seen as early as eight years after treatment.

When you *are* at increased risk: options for prevention

Many women at increased risk for developing breast cancer are interested to know what, if anything, they can do to reduce their risk. While there are many options for *treatment* of breast cancer, unfortunately the effective options for *prevention* are surprisingly limited.

1. Obesity and heavy alcohol consumption are two lifestyle factors that increase risk for breast cancer for *all* women (see chapter 13 for more on the topic of lifestyle factors), so avoiding these is definitely advisable for women already at increased risk.
2. Prophylactic or risk-reducing mastectomy (surgically removing the breasts) is typically reserved for those at highest risk for breast cancer, such as BRCA mutation carriers (see chapter 15).
3. Tamoxifen is a medication that is most commonly given to women *with* breast cancer as a treatment to reduce the risk of their cancer coming back (see chapter 9 for more on tamoxifen treatment). But tamoxifen is also approved as a preventive agent and prescribed for selected women who don't have breast cancer but who are at increased risk for developing it. In this group, tamoxifen reduces risk by approximately 50 percent. So, for example, women with LCIS who have a 20 percent lifetime risk of developing breast cancer can take tamoxifen, thereby reducing their overall risk to approximately 10 percent. Many assume that most women at increased risk for breast cancer, the majority of whom are understandably anxious about developing the disease, would enthusiastically take a medication that could reduce their risk so dramatically. Surprisingly, only a small percentage of those eligible for tamoxifen as a preventive agent actually do take it. In part this is due to physicians' lack of awareness: many general doctors are not familiar with the criteria that place a woman at increased risk, and therefore don't offer the drug to their patients who are eligible. But research also shows that even among eligible women who *are* offered

tamoxifen, only a minority take it. The majority of women who are at increased risk for breast cancer but otherwise generally healthy cite the fear of side effects as their main reason for being unwilling to take it. I do offer tamoxifen to my patients who are eligible and encourage them to take it. But for many the side effects are real and a source of concern, and I completely understand why some choose not to take it. Raloxifene (Evista) is another drug similar to tamoxifen that is an option for breast cancer prevention, but it is effective only in postmenopausal women. Evista was actually initially approved as an osteoporosis medication and is primarily prescribed for that indication. However, in a large breast cancer prevention trial comparing raloxifene to tamoxifen, raloxifene was found to have a preventive effect on breast cancer, although not as robustly as tamoxifen, but also was found to have a milder side effect profile as well. For postmenopausal women who have osteoporosis *and* are at increased risk for breast cancer, raloxifene can be a good option, killing two birds with one stone.

MYTH: "Having breast implants increases your risk of cancer *and* makes it harder to detect cancer on a mammogram."

Let me just say this plainly: breast implants *do not* increase one's risk of getting breast cancer, nor do they make it more difficult to detect breast cancer on mammograms. In most well-equipped and experienced radiology practices, the technicians are trained to get good views of the actual breast tissue by displacing the implants back toward the chest wall. It's worth keeping in mind that extra images are almost always routinely needed for women with breast implants, as extra views allow us to more fully visualize the breast tissue surrounding the implants on all sides. What is true is that breast implants *may* make it more difficult to do a needle biopsy of an abnormality if one is found on a mammogram. If the abnormality is deep in the breast, many radiologists are appropriately nervous about the puncture risk associated with sticking a long, sharp needle anywhere near the implant. In these cases, you may need surgery, which can remove the concerning area under direct visualization, with less risk of damaging the implant. An experienced breast radiologist will usually be able to guide you toward the appropriate procedure if you have implants and need a biopsy.

Mammograms and radiation exposure

Mammograms use radiation to create a picture of your breast tissue. Many women are understandably concerned about the amount of radiation an annual mammogram exposes them to (as well as the radiation from any associated tests required if the mammogram shows an abnormality). My answer to this is that concerns about radiation exposure from mammograms causing cancer are unwarranted and *not* a good excuse for opting out.

For one thing, it's important to know that we are exposed to radiation in day-to-day life, no matter what we do. For example, people who live at higher altitudes have increased radiation exposure over their lifetimes because there is less atmosphere to absorb sources of radiation from above. The same goes for people who take regular airplane flights. These small increases in radiation exposure are not significant enough to increase the risk of developing cancer for the vast majority of women—which is why people continue to live at high altitudes and fly in airplanes! The mammogram is associated with one of the lowest amounts of radiation exposure of any medical test, roughly the equivalent of ten long plane flights. By contrast, a CT scan of the lungs, such as might be recommended for lung cancer screening, is associated with more than twenty times the radiation exposure of a mammogram (or two hundred long plane flights).

Mammography and overdiagnosis

There is no question that as mammograms and other screening tools get better and better and identify more and more findings, in some cases cancer is being overdiagnosed and therefore overtreated. For example, there are many cancers that are small and slow-growing, and if not detected, they could percolate along for years before causing any harm whatsoever. A woman with one of these types of cancers may end up dying of some other, unrelated illness, and the only way we would find out that *incidentally* she had breast cancer is from an autopsy. It stands to reason that there's no point in treating these types of less threatening cancers.

However, at this point in time, we in the medical profession are not very good at distinguishing the life-threatening cancers from the ones that may just cruise along. Let me be clear: most cancers don't just cruise along. And so when we see a cancer, no matter how small or apparently insignificant, we typically treat it, knowing that the risk of no treatment would be losing the opportunity to cure a life-threatening cancer. One day we will have the tools to reliably tell the difference between a cancer we need to treat and a cancer that we don't, but we are not there yet. Much research is being done in this area, and I'm confident that in the future our tools for diagnosis will improve substantially. Until then, the mammogram remains our most reliable tool.

Screening Versus Diagnostic Tests

There are other tests that we can use to screen for breast cancer, specifically ultrasounds and MRIs, but the context in which we are administering the test is important. When talking about testing in general, it's necessary to distinguish between two types of test: screening and diagnostic.

1. Screening tests

A screening test is a fishing expedition of sorts. When a person has no identifiable or specific abnormalities that we are investigating, the test she undergoes is a screening test. So when a woman comes to my office for her annual checkup and has a mammogram, this is a screening test. If a woman has a normal mammogram and a normal physical exam and we want to do an ultrasound just to see if anything else can be found, it's a screening ultrasound.

2. Diagnostic tests

A diagnostic test is thought of as a targeted exam: it means something of concern has already been identified, and we want to get tests to figure out or diagnose exactly what is going on with the finding. So if a woman comes into my office after noticing a mass in her breast, then we would do a diagnostic mammogram and/or ultrasound.

Ultrasound: when to screen

For the vast majority of women, ultrasounds *alone* are not appropriate for early breast cancer detection, as they are not nearly as effective as mammograms. In fact, when the physical examination and mammogram are normal, screening ultrasound picks up only a very small percentage of additional cancers—1 to 2 percent in most women. Furthermore, even the most thorough ultrasound examination cannot give us a comprehensive and total picture of the whole breast the way a mammogram does, since the ultrasound probe allows us to visualize only one segment of the breast at a time, and spots can be missed.

In general, ultrasounds should be performed in selected patients *in addition* to mammograms as a screening test, or as a diagnostic test to get a better look at something already identified either by mammogram or because the patient or doctor feels something that seems new or abnormal. The risks and benefits of screening ultrasounds are variable based on the patient, and so, just like everything related to breast cancer, there is no one-size-fits-all recommendation. What we know for certain is that not all women need a screening ultrasound, and screening ultrasound is associated with an increased number of false positives, since the more you look, the more you find. Some of the factors that may influence your and your doctor's decision about whether to add an ultrasound to your screening include

- Having a higher risk for breast cancer related to some of the risk factors described above.
- Having dense breasts. Breast density becomes a factor when the normal tissue appears thicker, making it more difficult to pick up cancers against the normal background on mammograms. If you have dense breasts (based on results from your mammogram), screening ultrasound is often useful and recommended. Recently legislation has been passed in many states—starting in Connecticut and including California, Texas, New York, and others—requiring radiologists to inform patients of their breast density after a mammogram so that screening ultrasound can be discussed and added to the testing lineup. So you can certainly expect that ultrasounds will be offered to more women and discussed more frequently, be-

cause many states now mandate it. The degree of breast density is determined by the radiologist reading your mammogram, and classified based on a four-level scale:

1. Fatty: breast tissue is composed of primarily fatty tissue, not dense at all
2. Scattered areas of density: minimal amounts of dense tissue
3. Heterogeneously dense: significant amount of dense tissue seen in different parts of the breast
4. Extremely dense: dense tissue uniformly throughout the breast

As the extent of breast density goes up the scale, the more difficult it can be to see a cancer against the background of dense tissue, and therefore the more potential benefit of detecting a cancer that mammograms might miss by adding ultrasound to the screening regimen. If you live in a state where notification regarding breast density is mandated, and you do receive notification that your breasts are dense along with the results of your mammogram, ask the doctor who ordered the mammogram, "Should I also be getting an ultrasound? Might it be beneficial in my particular case?"

Ultrasound: what to expect

Unlike mammograms, ultrasounds do not involve radiation exposure, and are appealing for that reason. An ultrasound exam (also called sonogram) involves lying on your back on an exam table. Usually the ultrasound technician or the doctor puts some clear gel on the breast skin surface to allow the ultrasound probe to glide over the skin surface more easily and smoothly. The ultrasound probe is about six inches long and is usually the shape of an electric razor but with a smooth surface on its working end. The end of the probe is placed on the skin surface and moved methodically over the breast in circles until as much of the skin surface as possible has been covered. The ultrasound probe is actually transmitting harmless, painless sound waves through the skin, allowing us to see structures in the breast tissue. This permits us to differentiate between fluid (a cyst, for example) and solid (perhaps a tumor), and often shows us lumps that stand out from the surrounding normal breast tissue.

MRI: when to screen

Screening for breast cancer with MRI is also controversial, and currently it is recommended only for groups at significantly higher risk. Though MRI does not involve radiation, it is—like ultrasound—associated with a high rate of false positive findings, more than seen with mammograms, and is generally *not* recommended for screening in the general population at all. Even among those at elevated risk, current recommendations involve screening only those at *highest* risk. As a reminder, the highest-risk groups are those who are known or suspected BRCA mutation carriers, those who were treated with chest wall radiation at a young age, and those with a combination of risk factors that put them at a risk of 20 to 25 percent of getting breast cancer over their lifetimes.

For other risk groups, such as those with atypia or those at 15 to

20 percent risk (the mild to moderately elevated risk group), less is known about the benefits of MRI screening. And even for women who have already had breast cancer, the benefits of yearly MRI screening in detecting future recurrence or a new cancer in the other breast have not been clearly established.

As breast MRI is *not* a standard testing procedure for breast cancer, the decision to get one should not be made lightly. Instead, it needs to be based on your personal risk factors and the results from other imaging tests. Unless you are in a particularly high risk group, it's likely that an MRI could lead to an unnecessary biopsy, multiple follow-up MRIs, and other tests. This likelihood far outweighs the likelihood that MRI will find a cancer.

MRI: what to expect

MRI is an imaging test that can be performed on almost any part of the body. However, to get the best picture of the breast, special machinery and software are needed, and not all facilities have these critical additions. Certainly most specialized breast centers and major or academic medical centers will. If you are at a smaller facility, you may want to ask if they have an MRI machine dedicated to breast imaging. With MRI, you usually lie facedown in a big tube as you go through the MRI machine, and an injection of dye called gadolinium is given through an IV during the test to better differentiate cancer from normal tissue. The test takes approximately thirty to forty-five minutes. With MRI there is no radiation involved, only magnetic waves, which have no known side effect. There are very few known side effects of the gadolinium injection (occasionally there can be an allergic reaction to the gadolinium), but we don't know if it's safe during pregnancy, so it's not recommended for pregnant women. In addition, women who have certain kinds of metal implants in their bodies, such as pacemakers, usually cannot have MRIs because the magnetic force of the scan runs the risk of displacing any metal device secured in the body.

Lying down in a tube doesn't sound uncomfortable (unless you are having the MRI for a back issue or other orthopedic concern in which lying down itself is uncomfortable), but many people feel very claustrophobic. There are open MRI machines, but most of these open machines do not do a great job of looking at breast tissue. So getting an MRI if you feel anxious in closed or tight spaces could be a problem. But getting screened with MRI is a critical part of the screening regimen for those at the highest risk, and important to do if you fall into one of these groups. If an MRI is recommended for you but you are worried about the experience, speak to your doctor about strategies for relaxation, meditation, or even medication to get through it.

Cutting-edge screening and diagnostic tools

Not yet ready for prime time, but possibly coming soon

Many biotechnology companies are championing and promoting new, exciting techniques for breast cancer screening and detection. Some of these are interesting, but more work needs to be done to ascertain the ultimate benefit for most women. Here are some of the newer tests that are being used selectively at reputable breast centers across the country:

- For many years scientists have suggested that cancer cells generate more heat than normal cells. If this is the case, it may be possible that we can use thermography to detect subtle temperature differences in cells and therefore identify cancers. Thermography is offered as an experimental test in some centers. Interesting, but certainly not ready for prime time.

- There are newer tests that combine PET scanning with mammograms or MRIs. PET scanning examines how a suspicious area takes up glucose, because we know that tumors take up more glucose than normal tissue. This type of testing may help refine results, helping determine whether something seen on a mammogram or MRI is more or less likely to be cancer.

- BSGI, a test that looks at uptake of certain radioactive dyes by tumors, is being used in combination with standard imaging in many centers throughout the country. Much research is being done to try to define how it might help differentiate cancer from normal tissue and reduce false positive results on mammograms and MRIs.

Experimental breast imaging: a cautionary tale

A few years back, a test called ductal lavage attracted a lot of interest, and was actually being performed by a number of doctors in their offices. The idea behind the test is that you could draw fluid and cells from the breast through a needle inserted into the nipple, and these cells could give you information regarding a woman's risk for developing breast cancer in the future. It was believed that the same test could even tell you whether or not she had already developed the disease, even if the cancer could not be seen on other imaging tests. The problem with ductal lavage was that before it was put into practice, it was never fully evaluated in a way that reliably and scientifically determined the validity of the test's results. As a result, if a doctor performed the test and retrieved cells that looked like cancer, it was very hard to know what to do with this information. Was it possible that the woman did *not* actually have cancer? Yes. What was the likelihood of this? Not known. If the doctor performed the test and got cancer cells out, was it possible that the woman did have cancer? Yes. However, if the mammogram and other tests were normal, how would we find it? We can't. And if the doctor found nothing on these standard tests, then what? Not sure. Rarely did the physician actually performing the test (usually a primary care physician or gynecologist) know what to do with the test results or how to act on them if they were abnormal. So as quickly as ductal lavage came into practice, it fell out of favor, and it is generally not promoted or performed anymore by practitioners of any kind.

So if your doctor wants to perform a nonstandard or experimental test (in other words, any test other than mammogram, ultrasound, or MRI), you should find out exactly how he or she intends to deal with the results. When your physician proposes a new diagnostic test, you can simply ask the following questions: "What are the possible outcomes of this test? What will you do in each eventuality?" If the answer to the second question is "I'm not really sure, but I can send you to a breast specialist to figure it out," you probably should think twice and see the breast specialist for advice *before* you have the test. The reality is that experimental tests can open up a whole can of worms, leading to extensive amounts of additional unnecessary tests, biopsies, and anxiety—and even with all the additional testing, you may not receive a definitive, satisfying resolution. So be careful when starting down this path of additional tests of unknown significance. And never assume that there is no downside. Remember, more is not necessarily better.

Testing frequency: why screening more regularly doesn't necessarily lead to better results

If screening improves the chances of cancer being detected earlier, then many people make the leap to assuming that more frequent testing would be even better. Many patients ask me why I don't order mammograms for them two or three times a year. They would be willing to do it if it would reduce the chance of a cancer being missed. But in most cases, when a mammogram does miss a cancer, it's because the cancer just isn't seen on a mammogram *at all*, even when we know that it is actually there. This is the case with 10 to 15 percent of all breast cancers. Doing mammograms more frequently won't detect a cancer that can't be seen on a mammogram in the first place. Sad to say, no matter which screening regimen is appropriate for you, it must be understood that there is *no* test or combination of tests at any interval or frequency that can effectively *guarantee* early detection.

Interval cancers

Every now and again, a patient whose mammogram was normal the month before comes in because she feels a new lump. And then the lump turns out to be cancer. In these cases, patients are understandably upset. "I have been totally on top of my screening," they say. "How did the mammogram miss my cancer? What happened?" This can happen because, no matter how frequently exams (physical or radiologic) are performed, there are cancers that cannot be seen on imaging studies, some of which are biologically aggressive, that can develop. These are known as interval cancers. They are demoralizing to both doctor and patient, and shake the foundations of our belief that surveillance and close follow-up are our safeguards. Fortunately, these cases are rare. The good news is that appropriate screening *does* increase the likelihood of early detection, which leads to a higher likelihood of cure. And certainly these interval cancers are still as potentially treatable and curable as their mammographically detected counterparts.

A WORD TO THE WISE

When getting any breast imaging test—mammogram, sonogram, MRI—there are two things that factor into the quality of the exam: the caliber of the equipment and the expertise of the radiologist actually looking at and interpreting the results. While it's difficult for a layperson to evaluate the actual equipment, there are ways to make sure you are at a facility that delivers quality care. Here are some things to look for:

1. In 1992 Congress passed the Mammography Quality Standards Act (MQSA), aimed at improving and unifying the standards for facilities, personnel, and the practice of performing mammography across the country. Today, a facility requires actual U.S. Food and Drug Administration (FDA) approval to perform mammograms, and you should always make sure the facility where you are having your mammogram is FDA approved. The FDA website does have a list of almost nine thousand facilities across the country that are approved (see the list of online resources at the back of the book).

2. You increase the likelihood of getting state-of-the-art technology by going to a facility that does a large volume of breast imaging, such as a dedicated breast imaging center, and that has the capability to perform breast biopsies if necessary. Your breast radiology facility should definitely offer digital mammograms. If it doesn't, you can be sure it is behind the times.

3. When it comes to the physician, if at all possible make sure that it's a specialized breast radiologist who is reading your mammogram, sonogram, MRI, or other breast imaging test. Reading and interpreting these tests accurately (not missing a cancer if there is one and, conversely, not overcalling normal findings) is best done by specialists who are looking at high volumes of breast imaging tests every day and who have received specialty training in this field. Breast imaging and the technology involved are also constantly evolving and improving, and simply put, it's hard for a general radiologist to keep up. Clearly a general radiologist who is looking at a brain MRI one minute and a chest CAT scan the next cannot possibly have the same level of expertise as a spe-

cialist when looking at your mammogram. And if an abnormality is identified on your images, a specialized breast radiologist would usually be the best person to perform and interpret the follow-up studies and biopsy if necessary, which involves a very specific skill set and training. Most specialized breast radiologists have done advanced training in breast imaging, and most read a minimum of approximately two thousand mammograms a year to maintain their skills.

4. If it is the first time you are going to a new breast radiology facility and have had previous exams elsewhere, the new facility should insist that you bring prior images if at all possible. Every woman's "normal" mammogram pictures differ in subtle ways, and comparing your previous pictures to the new ones is a critical part of interpreting your imaging study results, whether it's a mammogram, sonogram, or MRI.

It's easy to find out if your facility is FDA approved, whether or not it offers digital mammograms, and who will be reading your mammogram. Just ask at the facility.

Self-examination

As with mammograms, there's been plenty of controversy and conflicting information surrounding the value of self-examination. Should women check themselves for lumps? How could there possibly be a downside to self-examination? The main downside, again, is the anxiety and fear generated by uncertainty. How do you know if you've found something irregular? If your breasts feel lumpy anyway, how can you tell if you've found something you should be worried about?

When it comes to self-examination, my recommendation is that it is always advisable for you to be familiar with your body and therefore aware of what is normal *for you*. In the same way that we consider it important for a woman to take notice when a new mole or dark spot has developed on her skin, it is critically important for you to have a basic idea of what's normal for your breasts so that if something new develops, you have a higher likelihood of noticing it.

That said, self-examination can be difficult, intimidating, and anxiety-provoking, especially if you are very lumpy and bumpy. But here's the deal: *every* woman's breasts can feel like a cobblestone street. Lumpy can be normal. And a woman's own exam can change over the course of the month related to her hormonal cycle as well. What you are looking for is a "dominant" finding or a change from what was previously there. And the only way to notice if there is a change in your breasts is to be somewhat familiar with what they feel like in the first place. Here are some signs to look for when you are looking for a new development:

- A mass in the breast that is new or larger than before. These features are more worrisome if the mass is firm and irregular.
- A new thickening in the breast. A thickening is less obvious than a mass, but it can feel as if there is a ridge of tissue in the breast. A thickening in the breast may be especially concerning if it is asymmetric when compared to the other breast.
- A subtle dimpling or indentation of the skin. These kinds of irregularities are often noticed when looking down at the skin, or seen on the undersurface of the breast when looking in the mirror. A dimpling can look as though the skin is being pulled inward by something beneath the skin's surface.
- Any change in the nipple, such as an inversion, hardening, scabbing, or flaking, especially if it's new or asymmetric to what you feel or see in the other breast.
- Nipple discharge, especially if it's bloody, and especially if it's only from one breast. Nipple discharge is also more concerning if it's spontaneous, meaning it comes out by itself rather than when the breast is squeezed. Spontaneous nipple discharge is commonly first noticed as a small stain in the bra or on pajamas. While there are also many noncancerous reasons for nipple discharge, new nipple discharge can be related to cancer and should be investigated.
- Changes to the breast skin color or thickness. New redness or thickening of the breast skin (so that it looks and feels leathery or like the skin of an orange), especially if not related to breast-

feeding or a known breast infection, is something that should be checked out.

- An enlarged or hard lump or lymph node in the armpit.

My advice is to examine your breasts once a month or so, but not obsessively. For women who menstruate, the best time each month is usually a week to ten days after you get your period. After a few cycles of self-exams, you'll likely become more comfortable and familiar with your baseline "normal" and less anxious overall.

THE TAKEAWAY

- For women without any identifiable risk factors, mammograms need to start at age forty.
- Mammograms may need to start earlier for those with a family history of breast cancer diagnosis at a young age.
- Ultrasounds can be done as an adjunct to mammograms for women at increased risk or with dense breasts.
- MRIs are for women at the highest risk for breast cancer.
- Regular self-exams are a good idea.
- Early detection is a goal, not a guarantee for anyone, no matter how diligent you are.

CHAPTER 2

Figuring Out if There Is a Problem and the "B" Word

when "We just need to take another look"

turns into a biopsy

At the age of fifty-two, Jennifer had gone for her annual mammogram at a local screening center. About a week later she received a letter in the mail: "Additional imaging and/or biopsy is needed." When she called the center directly to find out what this meant in plain English, they told her: "We found something. We need to take another look."

Whether a total surprise (after a routine annual) or something you sort of anticipated (because you yourself found a lump during self-examination), these are the words that no one wants to hear after a mammogram. But even so, when you *do* hear those words, remember that it may not be anything worrisome, and if it is, your doctor is doing his or her job. It's very important for us to know whether what's showing up on the mammogram is cancer or not. And the only way to know this is through further testing.

What to expect: follow-up testing

Usually the first step in investigating anything found on a mammogram is additional close-ups or magnification mammogram pictures of the area of concern. Often an ultrasound targeted to the area is done as well. Many women are understandably anxious to find out if there is truly any concern and want to come back in right away, and most radiology facilities are able to accommodate the need for follow-up examinations within a reasonable amount of time (a week). While many women who receive the news that they need follow-up can't get back in fast enough and feel as though even an extra day is too long to wait, it's important to know that it's not a medical emergency. Certainly you should return within a month to follow up. In the best-case scenario, this additional imaging completely resolves the concern; a lump turns out to be a simple cyst that is completely normal, or tissue that looked like a mass was found to be just two areas that were overlapping, making them look more dense and concerning on the original pictures. With these kinds of explanations—a cyst, overlap, dense tissue—your doctor will likely ask you to come back for your normal annual mammogram in a year. Sometimes follow-up is recommended at a shorter interval, usually six months, just to be on the safe side.

Then there are those cases when the additional pictures do confirm that there is something concerning. When this happens, a biopsy is usually the next step.

Next step: biopsy

At this point in your care, it is usually your primary care doctor or gynecologist (the doctor who ordered your mammogram) and the breast radiologist who are your point people, discussing your results with you and making recommendations about next steps. Occasionally at the first sign of concern you will be referred to a breast surgeon, who can weigh in even at this early point, when results may turn out to be completely normal. In any case, when a concerning finding has been identified on your physical examination, an imaging study, or both, a biopsy is usually recommended.

In general, there are two ways a biopsy can be done: a needle biopsy or a surgical biopsy.

Needle biopsy: what to expect

A needle biopsy usually involves the use of local anesthetic (injected into the overlying skin) or topical anesthetic (applied to the skin surface) and is done in the breast radiology facility or center. There are several types of needle biopsy, defined by the type of technology that's being used to guide the needle.

- A *stereotactic* or *mammotome core biopsy* is a needle biopsy that is performed while you are in the mammogram machine, using the actual mammogram pictures for guidance. The breast is compressed, and usually a technician and a breast radiologist guide the needle to the area of interest. I know, it sounds like nothing could feel worse: having your breast squashed in a mammogram machine *and* also having a needle stuck into it at the same time! But they do give you local anesthesia, and a skilled physician and technician will work quickly to do the procedure as accurately and as fast as possible.
- An *ultrasound-guided core biopsy* is a needle biopsy that is performed while you are having an ultrasound, using the ultrasound for guidance.
- An *MRI-guided core biopsy* is a needle biopsy that is performed while you are in the MRI machine, using the actual MRI images for guidance.

The above three are essentially the same procedure, using the same general type of needle. The main difference is just the kind of imaging test being used to guide the biopsy needle to the right spot. In the best-case scenario, it is a specialized breast radiologist who performs these image-guided procedures. In some cases, breast surgeons receive training in biopsy techniques and perform these procedures in offices equipped with the necessary machinery (mammogram or sonogram), especially in smaller cities and towns where specialized radiology practices and services may not be as widely available.

The whole process takes anywhere from fifteen to thirty minutes, including proper positioning and preparing the imaging, but the actual needle-sticking part usually takes less than five minutes. A small nick in the skin is made and tiny snippets of tissue are removed from the targeted area. There can be some soreness and bruising after a biopsy, but there is very little scarring internally, and almost no residual skin scar other than the small needle stick site. Occasionally, some bad bruising will occur but this is uncommon, and will resolve on its own. Recovery after needle biopsy is instantaneous and most patients are back to their usual routine the next day.

- A *fine needle aspiration,* also called an *FNA,* uses a skinnier needle that gets out only a small sample of cells and not actual pieces of tissue the way a core biopsy does. This type of biopsy is frequently performed when a surgeon feels something concerning in the breast or in a lymph node and does an FNA through the skin directly overlying the abnormality. While FNA can be done in your doctor's office and is a quick procedure, the results are usually not as definitive or clear-cut as those provided by one of the core biopsy techniques described above. The reason for this is that FNA only gets a small sample of breast cells, not actual tissue. Some surgeons are unwilling to operate based on FNA results alone, so you might need to get a core biopsy as well.

Surgical biopsy: what to expect

Surgical biopsy is a much more invasive procedure than needle biopsy. As the name suggests, it involves actual surgery. While it is possible to perform a surgical biopsy using local anesthetic alone, in most cases patients are sedated with intravenous anesthesia, and therefore the biopsy is most often done in a hospital or outpatient surgery setting. The procedure takes approximately thirty to forty-five minutes and involves an incision made in the skin of the breast, removal of a sample of the suspicious area, and closure with stitches. This small surgery does not involve an overnight stay and is usually performed as a day surgery procedure, but some women do take time off from work for a day or more because of soreness and bruising in the breast. Recovery time is longer than with the needle biopsy, and if your job involves any upper-body activity such as lifting or carrying, you will probably need a week or more of rest before you can return to work. It's best to hold off on rigorous exercise for that period too. With a surgical biopsy there is almost always some residual scar that can be seen, although these scars can usually be strategically placed to minimize their prominence—for example, around the edge of the areola (the darker-colored skin around the nipple), where the color change hides the incision.

When possible, needle biopsy is best

In general, needle biopsies are much less invasive, involving much less recovery time and less scar formation than a surgical biopsy. In the vast majority of cases when an experienced, technically adept professional performs a needle biopsy, the results are clear and conclusive and obtained less invasively. As a general rule, if information and results can be obtained accurately with a smaller, less invasive procedure, this is the way to go. In addition, if the needle biopsy results are normal and conclusive—and frequently they are—then surgery can be avoided altogether.

Another advantage of a needle biopsy is that results can usually be obtained within a day or two of the procedure. If results show cancer, the diagnosis can be made *before* performing any surgery at all. You and your doctor can then sit down, discuss results, and make plans for surgery knowing more about what your diagnosis is and what your options are. With a surgical biopsy, the patient undergoes an operation, albeit a small one, to remove something in the breast. The results are obtained a few days later, usually longer than it takes to get needle biopsy results. When the results come back showing cancer, the conversation regarding appropriate next steps happens *after* this first surgery is already done, and almost always requires more surgery. Thus the number of operations required can often be minimized by using a needle biopsy first, to get critical information about what is going on, before any surgery is performed.

When a needle biopsy is not possible

There are certainly circumstances where a needle biopsy *cannot* be performed and where you will need a surgical biopsy. Here's the list of those possible scenarios:

- Some locations in the breast (either very superficial or very deep, for example) are not accessible with the needle.
- It can be extremely difficult to perform needle biopsies on women with very small breasts. When a small breast is being compressed in a mammogram machine for a stereotactic biopsy, for instance, a needle could go right through the breast and miss the target completely.
- Women with breast implants may often require surgical biopsies, as radiologists may be hesitant to stick a needle into the breast and possibly damage or rupture the implant.
- Women with certain conditions that prevent them from lying still in the position required for a needle biopsy for a long enough period of time may require surgical biopsy. This may include women with a bad back, a movement disorder such as Parkinson's disease or cerebral palsy, or women who have difficulty breathing when lying flat (this can be due to a variety of reasons, including congestive heart failure or obesity).
- When your doctor feels a mass in your breast, yet all imaging studies are normal, a needle biopsy really can't be done guided

by imaging, since the imaging didn't show anything in the first place. Even when the mammogram and ultrasound are completely normal, a suspicious mass can *still* be a cancer and should be further investigated. In these rare cases, your surgeon may want to take it out surgically just to make sure a cancer is not being missed.

A WORD TO THE WISE

If your surgeon recommends you have a surgical biopsy and you *don't* fall into one of the categories listed above, you may want to seek a second opinion. Some surgeons, especially those who are *not* breast specialists, favor surgical biopsies without adequate justification. There have been various studies showing that in certain geographical areas, such as rural areas or areas without breast specialists, far too many surgical biopsies are being performed, and patients who are eligible for needle biopsies are not being appropriately referred for them with enough frequency. While surgical biopsies should be done no more than 10 percent of the time, one study from Florida showed that up to 30 percent of biopsies were done surgically. This may be because a surgeon can make more money from a surgical biopsy, or it may be because the area lacks doctors with expertise in performing needle biopsies. Recent studies also have shown that surgeons who do not receive specialty training—and therefore may not have the highest level of understanding of the best practices for diagnosis of breast cancer—are more likely to recommend a surgical biopsy than to appropriately refer a patient to a radiologist for a needle biopsy. Again, if your surgeon insists you have a surgical biopsy and you don't fall into one of the categories listed above, you may want to seek a second opinion.

MYTH: "Needle biopsies spread cancer."

Somehow, at some point, someone came up with the misinformation that needle biopsies can spread cancer—and if a needle biopsy is done and shows cancer, surgery needs to be done quickly thereafter to contain the cancer and reduce the risk of spread caused by the needle. This is simply not true! The needle biopsy is a critical tool in diagnosis of breast cancer and many other cancers in other organs of the body. Most important, it does not spread cancer. While there are minimal risks associated with the needle biopsy, including bleeding and infection, cancer spread is *not* one of them. So please don't refuse the needle biopsy because of concern about the possibility of cancer spread.

Marking the spot

If you are having a needle biopsy, your radiologist or sometimes the surgeon performing the biopsy should plan on leaving a marker in the area of concern. A marker is a tiny metallic clip, usually made of titanium, which can be seen on future mammograms. The clips also come in different shapes (there's a ribbon shape that looks like a tiny version of the pink breast cancer ribbon, an hourglass shape, a top hat shape, and others) so that if more than one biopsy is performed, different shapes can be used to demarcate the different spots. There is no reason to refuse to let the radiologist put in the marker. Markers are harmless and painless, and if you are diagnosed with a small cancer, it will make it infinitely easier for your surgeon to zero in and find exactly the right spot.

Oftentimes when a needle biopsy is done, the area that is being biopsied is quite small. So small, in fact, that the needle biopsy alone can remove the whole area. For example, one of the most common findings leading to a biopsy is the identification of new microcalcifications on a mammogram. Microcalcifications are tiny white specks that look like grains of salt on the mammogram. When a patient has her yearly mammogram and new calcifications are seen, biopsy is usually recommended. Calcifications can involve the entire breast or a very limited area, as small as a few tiny dots over a quarter of an inch. When a biopsy is performed, the needle is inserted multiple times, coring out a small area of tissue containing the calcifications. When the area undergoing biopsy is tiny to begin with, the entire extent of calcifications that are seen may be removed by the biopsy alone. A few days after the biopsy is done, the pathology report comes back. Of all calcifications that undergo biopsy, approximately 20 percent will be cancerous. If the results do show cancer, the doctor may no longer be able to precisely find the area on the mammogram if the tiny calcifications were completely removed. But it is important to realize that just because the calcifications have been removed or can no longer be seen, it does *not* necessarily mean that all the cancer has been removed! You will still need surgery to remove the surrounding area, and commonly there *is* still some cancer in the surrounding tissue even when it appears that the whole area of calcifications was removed during the biopsy. So the marker left at the time of the biopsy is the only way for the surgeon to know where to go.

Even with large cancers, clips can still be critical. For example, in some cases chemotherapy is given first to treat the cancer, and the cancer shrinks significantly. Without a clip marking the spot, the surgeon may not be able to find his or her way back to the right area to remove it. (For more on chemotherapy before surgery, see chapter 9.)

NEED TO KNOW

The markers that are left behind after biopsy are very small; they cannot be felt and cause no discomfort. Even if the biopsy result is normal and the area and the marker do not need to be removed, there is no harm having it in your breast permanently. The marker also won't cause you to set off any alarms in the airport, so you don't have to worry about being strip-searched next time you go on vacation (not because of the marker, anyway).

What a needle biopsy can tell you

A needle biopsy takes out small snippets of tissue from the area of concern. If the area of concern is very small, sometimes a significant portion of the area is removed just by the biopsy alone. If the area is larger, only a small part of the overall area is removed. Regardless of how big the area of concern is, the tissue removed by the needle biopsy usually provides an accurate representation of what is going on in that area. Results from the needle biopsy can be put into one of three categories:

1. Benign, or normal
2. Malignant, or cancer
3. Indeterminate (or as I tell my patients, "in-between")

Benign and malignant results usually provide us surgeons with the most important information regarding what we are dealing with and the direction we need to take. For normal results, often no further intervention is needed. For cancer, we sit down and talk about next steps. When a needle biopsy shows cancer, here's what it can tell you:

1. Whether your cancer is DCIS (noninvasive) or invasive. (See chapter 5 for more on types of cancer.)
2. If it's invasive, whether it's ductal cancer, lobular cancer, or some other unusual subtype. (Again, see chapter 5 for more on these particular types of cancer.)
3. The factors that are making the cancer grow. The needle biopsy can tell us whether or not the tumor is hormonally sensitive and dependent on the hormones estrogen and progesterone to help it grow and spread (see chapter 8 for further discussion). The needle biopsy can also give us information about Her2/neu status. Approximately 20 percent of breast cancers are Her2/neu-positive, and this can be important information to guide the course of treatment (also described in chapter 8).

A WORD TO THE WISE

For certain types of tumors, important decisions regarding the *order* of treatments can be made based on the biopsy results. For example, patients with triple negative (estrogen-, progesterone-, and Her2/neu-negative) or Her2/neu-positive cancers are sometimes considered for chemotherapy *before* surgery. (For more on chemotherapy before surgery, see chapter 9.) So it's important that these tests are performed on the biopsy specimen and discussed up front. If your tumor is triple negative or Her2/neu-positive, ask your surgeon if you should be seeing an oncologist before proceeding with surgery to help make those decisions.

What a needle biopsy can't tell you

Needle biopsies do have some limitations. For example, they usually cannot tell us the stage of the cancer—only surgery can do that. During the biopsy, we take only a small snippet of the tumor out, so we don't know the exact size of the whole tumor or whether or not the tumor has spread to the lymph nodes, which is key information for assessing the stage. And a needle biopsy can't always tell us the exact extent or amount of cancer in the breast. As a result, we can't always make decisions regarding what kind of surgery to recommend based on just a single biopsy result. Instead, we factor in other information to help guide us, including sometimes additional biopsies of other areas in the breast or the other breast. The need for additional biopsies or imaging before surgery is usually determined by your surgeon.

In approximately 10 percent of cases we will get indeterminate results from a biopsy. The indeterminate category includes instances when we didn't get enough tissue out to fully assess the area of concern, or when we see abnormal cells in the tissue removed, such as atypical cells, which occasionally live in the neighborhood of cancer. In these cases, we often proceed to surgery so we can take out a larger sample to get a clearer idea of what is going on, and to make sure we don't miss a cancer in the surrounding area. When results are indeterminate on the needle biopsy and we proceed with removing the surrounding area, the tissue we remove gets analyzed in the lab in the days after surgery. In about 10 to 20 percent of cases, we will find actual cancer in that surrounding tissue, which then sometimes requires additional surgery or treatment. Some women do say, "Well, if the area has to come out anyway, why should I have the needle biopsy to begin with? Who wants two procedures, a needle biopsy and then surgery, when you can have one?" The truth is most needle biopsies *do* give definitive results, benign or malignant, and indeterminate results are much less common. And of course there is no way to know prior to the procedure what the results will be. So concern about the unlikely scenario of receiving an indeterminate result is usually not a good reason to refuse needle biopsy in favor of going straight to surgery. For most women, the needle biopsy alone will get the job of definitive diagnosis done.

Another reason for biopsy: a new or enlarging lump

A new or enlarging lump in your breast is always a significant cause of concern, but there are a variety of different reasons you might have developed a lump, and many of those reasons are *not* cancer.

Not all lumps are cancer

The common causes of benign breast lumps include

- **Cysts.** Cysts are fluid-filled sacs that are typically very well rounded and can be any size. Many premenopausal women get breast cysts, and cysts can fluctuate with the menstrual cycle, becoming most pronounced right before a woman gets her period. Cysts can usually be differentiated from solid masses by ultrasound. Simple cysts are almost always normal and can be left alone. If there is any concern or discomfort related to the cyst (they can be tender sometimes), it can be aspirated with a needle, and it will usually disappear after that. Cysts can recur even after aspiration, but this does not necessarily indicate a problem, nor does recurrence indicate the need for surgical removal.
- **Benign masses.** When a mass or lump is solid (not a fluid-filled cyst) there is still a possibility that it is benign or normal, particularly in premenopausal women. One of the most common causes of a benign breast mass is a *fibroadenoma,* and many young women get them, even as early as their teenage years. *Fibrocystic disease,* which sounds scary (any condition with the word "disease" in its name can't be good, right?), is really just a description of the combination of normal lumps, bumps, and cysts in the breast that most women develop or experience at some point. However, for women of all ages, *any* new or enlarging solid breast lump must be tested for cancer until proven otherwise.

When your mammogram and ultrasound are normal, but your doctor says you need a biopsy anyway

"I'm off the hook, right?" Beth said to me hopefully.

"Unfortunately, no," I answered. Beth, a patient in her early forties, had identified a new lump high up in her left breast while in the shower one day. Her primary care doctor ordered a mammogram and an ultrasound. Both were normal. This was great news. However, because any unexplained new lump is concerning until proven not to be cancer, the doctor asked me to examine Beth in the hope of providing reassurance that nothing more needed to be done. Even without seeing Beth, I suspected something *would* need to be done. Any unexplained lump warrants explanation, and while it's true that a normal mammogram and ultrasound of the area do decrease the likelihood that the lump is cancerous, they do not eliminate the possibility. In general, a new lump usually requires a biopsy of some sort to get more definitive information regarding the nature of the lump, even when the ultrasound and mammogram are both normal.

When your surgeon recommends removing a noncancerous lump

There are some situations where, even if a needle biopsy shows normal findings, your doctor may still recommend removing the lump with surgery, especially if it's a larger mass. If you are planning on having children anytime soon, your doctor may recommend that the mass be removed before you do so. When you're pregnant, many lumps, even normal ones, will get larger due to hormonal stimulation, and this could lead to the highly undesirable situation of trying to decide whether you need surgery for an enlarging breast mass, which would expose mother and fetus to anesthesia and its associated risks. Therefore, a surgeon may well recommend surgical removal of a lump in a younger woman as a preemptive strike.

If the mass is not removed, your doctor should insist on reexamining you in two to three months to assess for changes. Clearly, if the mass goes away by itself, the problem is solved. Cancers, in general, do not spontaneously disappear, or even wax and wane. But any mass that persists or—more concerning—gets larger within the two- to three-month period should probably be removed at that point. Furthermore, if your lifestyle makes follow-up difficult (you are heading out to trek in Tibet for the next nine months, for example, or you have a job that makes it impossible for you to keep doctor's appointments), removal may be advisable from the start.

MYTH: "If there's a lump, it needs to come out no matter what."
Many women assume that if they feel a lump, or if we see a suspicious area on a mammogram or ultrasound, it needs to come out no matter what. Therefore they refuse needle biopsy in favor of surgery to remove the lump entirely. But the current standard of care is to perform a needle biopsy first, and no surgeon should recommend just taking out a suspicious mass without doing a needle biopsy (unless there is a good reason that a needle biopsy cannot be done—see "When a Needle Biopsy Is Not Possible").

A WORD TO THE WISE

If your doctor tells you that the new lump you feel or the new area he or she can see on your mammogram requires no further investigation or follow-up, you may want to get a second opinion to confirm that this is actually the case. No matter how innocuous a lump may seem, in most cases the only way to *prove* that it's benign is to perform a biopsy.

A WORD TO THE WISE

Many doctors who are *not* breast specialists make the mistake of "watching and waiting" to see if a mass changes before proceeding with even a needle biopsy, especially with younger women. The problem with this approach is that you might end up "watching and waiting" while a cancer grows. You don't have to drop everything to get a biopsy done; breast cancer doesn't grow over the course of days or weeks. But waiting more than one or two months with no further testing is not recommended, and the priority should be making sure that a cancer diagnosis isn't missed or delayed (another reason to have a breast cancer specialist in your corner). Nonspecialist surgeons sometimes argue that it is disfiguring to perform a "big operation" to obtain a biopsy. But nothing can be further from the truth. Again, needle biopsies are a minor procedure leaving virtually no scar and requiring only local anesthetic. Even when an operation is required to remove the lump, a breast surgeon will know how to minimize the incision—both in size and prominence of location— and will walk the fine line between removing enough to get rid of the mass and to provide a definitive result and not significantly altering the size or contour of the breast.

THE TAKEAWAY

- Whenever possible, choose a needle biopsy over surgery.
- A lump may still need a biopsy even if a mammogram and ultrasound are normal.
- With a needle biopsy, leaving behind a marker is key.

CHAPTER 3

When "Positive" Is a Negative Thing

the first steps to take when cancer is diagnosed

At age sixty-one, Wendy was conscientious about getting her yearly mammogram. She had a family history of breast cancer and also saw me for yearly examinations as part of our center's program for women at increased risk for breast cancer. She usually made the appointment for the day after her birthday. She reasoned that if it was good news and she got a normal mammogram report, then this was a birthday gift to herself. If it *wasn't* good news, at least it wouldn't ruin her birthday celebration.

One year Wendy's mammogram showed a new small cluster of white dots, called calcifications. I recommended that she have a biopsy, and she agreed. The results showed an early, small ductal carcinoma in situ, or DCIS. Of course, the only word Wendy heard when I gave her the diagnosis was "carcinoma," or cancer, and thus she assumed the worst.

"What does this mean?" she asked me nervously.

The first thing I told her was that although I would never tell a woman who was diagnosed with cancer that she was lucky, among all the possible types of cancer out there, DCIS is one that is very treatable and curable, and that's what I intended to do.

I also told Wendy to keep the following in mind:

1. **Stay calm (if you can).** For most women, the reaction to a breast cancer diagnosis is understandably one of shock, concern, and even panic. But it's important to try to find some way to feel hopeful and optimistic too. Cure rates for breast cancer have never been better. When breast cancer is detected early, survival rates can be higher than 90 percent, and in cases of DCIS, like Wendy's, survival can be as high as 98–99 percent. If at all possible, try to remain calm. Working with doctors who instill this sense of calmness and confidence in your prognosis will help; right from the start, don't choose any doctor who doesn't make you feel this way, who does not explain next steps in a way that makes sense to you, or who does not allot you enough time to answer all of your questions. Finding some sense of calmness comes with many benefits—after all, no one finds it easy to make important decisions under extreme amounts of duress. As you move forward, a calmer state of mind will allow you to process information, think more clearly, and make better decisions for yourself about your care.

2. **Remember, you are not in an emergency situation.** The only forgiving thing about a diagnosis of breast cancer is that it usually does not constitute a medical emergency. Breast cancer is not like appendicitis or a bowel obstruction, where you need to act within hours or else risk dire consequences. While many patients have visions of the cancer running wild and spreading throughout the body even in the time it takes to read an article in your doctor's waiting room or the pages in this book, the fact is that even the most aggressive newly diagnosed cancer does not grow or spread in a day, a week, or even a month; it takes a much longer period of time. Taking a week or two to consider your first steps and to arrange appointments with the right doctors in the best places, rather than taking the first appointment with whomever you can get, will not jeopardize a good outcome in any way. This does not mean you should delay treatment for too long. Once you've identified your plan of action (which the next few chapters will help you do), there's really no reason to wait. All that said, waiting can prolong the psychological agony. Ideally,

you want your surgery or treatment to begin within four to six weeks of diagnosis.

3. **It's not your fault.** It's important to know that you did not give yourself breast cancer, the way obesity can give you diabetes or smoking can give you lung cancer. Yes, there are some factors that can increase the risk of getting breast cancer (for more on this, see chapter 13), but even when these exist, they're usually not the only reasons. With all the complex emotions associated with a breast cancer diagnosis, guilt should not be one of them.

Involving others: sharing widely versus keeping the circle tight

At some point, everyone facing a breast cancer diagnosis will spend some time thinking about whom they want to tell about it and whom they would like to be involved in their treatment and recovery. The number of people you wish to be involved is really up to you. Before I operate, I always ask my patient, "Who is here with you today in the waiting room whom I can speak to when we are done with surgery?" Some patients have a veritable entourage of people camped out in the waiting room, anxiously awaiting any news I can give them. Some women have just their husband, their significant other, or a good friend or neighbor, not wanting to "bother" too many others (if this sounds like you, I will say that you'd be surprised by the number of people who are willing to help if you do decide to share the news more widely). Some people live relatively solitary, private existences and don't want to involve too many others in their lives, and sometimes people just don't have many people in their lives that they feel are close enough to involve. There is no one "right" answer—you are entitled to tell as many or as few people as you'd like.

If you are lucky enough to be surrounded by people who love you and who all want to take part in your care (and if you are willing to let those people into your confidence), remember there are advantages and disadvantages to having a larger number of people extensively involved.

The case for sharing widely

The benefits of involving a wider network of people are obvious: you'll have a more extensive support system to make sure you feel loved and cared for during your treatment and recovery. Some people in your life are uniquely qualified to be involved in your care and decision making. A husband, partner, or significant other should definitely have some role in helping figure out what's best for you, both as an individual and as part of a couple. A best friend or sibling might know things about your personality that may help in decision making as well.

The people that you *do* want fully involved should accompany you to consultations, ask questions, and be your advocate. When you are diagnosed with breast cancer and you meet with a doctor for the first time, it can be hard to process all the information you're hearing. In this situation, friends and family members can act as an extra set of ears, taking notes and reviewing them with you later. These loved ones can be excellent sounding boards as well. Most important, they remind you that although you may be the one with the diagnosis, you are not alone.

It can be incredibly moving to see how many people come out to help after a diagnosis of breast cancer. Whether it's extended family, friends, work colleagues, fellow congregants, or community members, it's often amazing how many people will find ways to step in and provide assistance and support with everything from school runs for the kids to stocking the fridge with home-cooked meals and or praying for you at church when you can't be there to do it yourself. These acts of kindness can be incredibly inspiring and endearing, and they seem to make the case that the more people that are involved, the better. Even so, it can be good to weigh the advantages of involving a lot of people against the disadvantages.

The case for keeping the circle tight

Keep in mind that the more people you tell, the more people you're going to have throwing in their two cents on your diagnosis and treatment. "My sister had breast cancer last year. You have to see her doctor!" "Make sure you don't get a needle biopsy; I've heard they spread cancer." "I had breast cancer. Make sure you get a lumpectomy—it's much less traumatic than a mastectomy." Although all these people mean well, they are likely *not* breast cancer experts and therefore should *not* be guiding your medical decisions. Breast cancer diagnosis and treatment are highly individualized, and what worked for one woman doesn't necessarily work for another. So when people in your circle want to provide information about your situation by drawing on their own sources, or when they start asking too many questions or getting involved in unproductive ways, it's fine to take a step back. My advice is to be grateful that people want to help, but to take these suggestions with a large pinch of salt, as there's a substantial chance that their information simply isn't relevant to you or, if based on their own experience years ago, possibly outdated.

Another note of caution: As a surgeon, I am always wary of the relative or friend who swoops in on the day of the operation and begins questioning the plan that's already in place, especially when I have never met that person at prior office visits. Sometimes this is a relative who lives out of town and can only be there for the surgery. Sometimes it is someone who just needs to feel involved in your life and make a contribution. In most cases, this last-minute arrival may prove confusing for you, undermining for the caregivers who have been there all along, and distracting to your surgeon. Family dynamics can be complicated, and a family member diagnosed with breast cancer inevitably brings up lots of issues for everyone. My advice is to remember that you are in charge, and to set ground rules and limits for those you choose to involve in your care at every stage.

What to tell your kids

When it's a mother receiving a breast cancer diagnosis, nine times out of ten her first thought is for her children. How will this affect the kids, particularly the younger ones? How can the impact on the children be minimized? And most urgently, what's the best way to tell them the news? Every mom wants to be there for her family, both now and in the long term, and so ensuring a rapid return to health becomes of paramount importance; often it's the only thing she can think about when diagnosed. If asked, I do have some age-appropriate guidelines for my patients about how to discuss what's going on with younger members of the family. The caveat, of course, is that I don't know your individual child or children. Ultimately only you know what's truly best for you and your family.

For all ages

Regardless of the age of the child, my advice is the same: if at all possible, don't overshare. There's no need to tell the children the minute you walk out of the doctor's office. Instead, it can be good to wait until a clear plan of action is in place so that you can communicate with your child confidently and from a place of calmness. Children of all ages need to feel that you are in control of the situation so that they can feel safe and secure.

Under age five

Children in this age group have little if any capacity to understand what a cancer diagnosis means. Even if your four-year-old daughter is super-smart and can count to a hundred in three languages, in all likelihood she won't be able to absorb the concept of breast cancer. In other words, your child doesn't need to know specifics about your current situation, as these will likely be confusing. What your child really needs to know is how your diagnosis will affect *him or her.* Will there be any major disruption to her schedule, your availability, or your appearance? It's best to hold off on saying too much too soon. Once surgery is scheduled and imminent, then you can decide what you feel your child absolutely needs to know. If he or she is three to five years old, you should definitely explain if you are staying in the hospital for a night or more: "Mommy needs to go to the hospital for one night this week. Grandma will take care of you, and you will have a great sleepover with her." If you speak to your child in simple, concrete terms about how your treatment and recovery will affect her day-to-day life, your child will likely feel strong and better able to cope.

In addition, my advice with this age group is to focus on the present and the immediate future. For example, if the need for chemotherapy cannot be determined at the time of diagnosis (as is often the case), then children in this age group do not need to hear, "Mommy may lose some hair next month." In fact, your child probably won't remember this information a month later. Better to wait until you have definite information to share and *then* communicate this to your child.

Five to eleven years old

Children in this age group have a significantly greater capacity to understand, absorb, and remember what you tell them, but again, they are usually most concerned about how a situation will affect *them*. Do your best to explain in simple, concrete terms any absences on your part or necessary changes to their schedules. If your appearance is going to change (for more on hair loss, see chapter 9 on chemotherapy and its side effects), you will need to prepare your child for that. Use of the word "cancer" needs to be considered very carefully. For many children, the word "cancer" means death, and this is about as far from the truth as possible for most women with breast cancer.

Remember that children in this age group are extremely sensitive and can pick up when you are feeling fearful and uncertain, which may cause them additional stress or confusion. Regardless of your prognosis and your own feelings, try your best to remain optimistic and upbeat when with your child. If things become more serious, children can be eased into these explanations and discussions as needed.

If you are planning on sharing the news with other adults in your life, you may want to tell your child first. It's always going to be better for your child to hear this news from you, rather than find out accidentally from a neighbor or another relative. Nowadays, many children in this age group have access to their own electronic devices or use their parents' devices or computers. With emails, texts, and cellphone messages flying back and forth, be careful that your child doesn't see or hear something before you're able to explain what's happening on your own terms. When you do have a plan in place, speak to your child with a tone of confidence about your well-being, regardless of how you really feel.

As much as possible, it's a good idea to leave children in this age group at home during your doctor's visits, as many children may find the experience upsetting. Of course, there are extenuating circumstances, especially when child care options are limited—for some women, if they can't bring their children to the appointment, they'll miss the appointment and won't get the care they need, which could have dire implications for the family beyond an upsetting (or boring) wait or conversation at the doctor's office.

Twelve to seventeen years old

Children in this age group are mature enough to understand what you are telling them about your diagnosis. However, what and how you tell them can still have an impact on them, so it's important to have a plan in place before you do share, so that everyone feels confident and secure.

While you are going through different parts of your treatment, most children at this age should be encouraged to go to school regularly, attend their usual activities, and maintain their usual schedules. Of course, this may not always be possible, and at times you may have to call on other family, friends, or community members to step in and provide support. Occasionally I'll see patients who bring teenage children with them to their appointments, expecting them to play the role of caregivers, and I often wonder if asking these kids to provide adult-level support to their parents is putting too much pressure on them. This "parentification," where the child assumes the role of the caretaker or adult, can be extremely stressful for a child. But some families do not have many options, and so having a child with them may be an important source of comfort (or simply logistically necessary). Many clinics or breast cancer centers have social workers available to help you with these issues, and even to entertain your child while you are in the appointment.

Keep in mind that your daughters in this age group may be particularly sensitive to discussions about breast cancer, and will naturally wonder about their own future risk. You can reassure your teenage daughter by telling her that there is almost no risk to her *at this point,* and while having a mother with breast cancer can increase her risk of developing breast cancer later in life, by then options for prevention and treatment will be even better than they are today.

Over eighteen years old

Children in this age group are essentially adults and may already be living away from home. Even so, when you first tell them you have breast cancer, they're still likely to feel fearful and insecure. Every day in my practice I see parents grappling with decisions about how and when to tell their adult children. Do you wait to tell the college student until after final exams, or the bride-to-be until after her wedding? What about the son or daughter who is in the military and deployed overseas—will he or she be distracted or endangered if told? There are no easy answers for any of these. With this age group, however, you can feel confident that you know your child better than anyone else does and that you will be able to come up with the best course of action for all concerned. Again, it's often beneficial to have some kind of plan in place before sharing. Although you wouldn't want to keep your adult children in the dark for too long, as this could lead to trust issues, it can be very distressing for children of any age to hear this type of news if you are still in turmoil yourself.

THE TAKEAWAY

- As much as possible, try to remain calm.
- As much as possible, try to maintain optimism.
- The news of your diagnosis should be shared in your own way and at your own pace, and with the right number of people for *you*.

CHAPTER 4

Putting Together Your Team

it starts with the surgeon

For most women, their primary care doctor, gynecologist, or breast radiologist has been spearheading their care and advising decision making up to this point. Once you are diagnosed with breast cancer, a different set of doctors will be needed to direct your care.

Most women diagnosed with breast cancer assume that right off the bat they need to see an oncologist. Oncologists are the doctors who take care of patients with cancer, right? Correct, but we need to qualify what we mean by an oncologist. In fact, there are three types of oncologists: surgical, medical, and radiation. Breast cancer care is multi-disciplinary. That means that different doctors from different disciplines of medicine (breast surgery, medicine, radiation, plastic and reconstructive surgery, and others) may be involved in different aspects of your care. And just to make it potentially more complicated, the number and types of different doctors and specialists that may be involved will vary from person to person and from case to case. Not *all* women need to see *all* these different types of doctors, and the order in which you see them may vary. Your particular case may require you to see a surgeon and then a medical oncologist, whereas your friend needed a medical oncologist, *then* a surgeon, and then a radiation oncologist. Given that most aspects of breast cancer care are sequential, not simultaneous, each doctor will be the "team captain" for that portion of your care, passing the baton to the next caregiver at the appropriate point for the next part of your treatment. While navigating the path through breast cancer treatment may seem particularly confusing and overwhelming, it's not. You just need to take the first step, and for most women newly diagnosed with breast cancer, the first step is to see the breast surgeon, or surgical oncologist. Almost all women who are newly diagnosed with breast cancer will have surgery as part of their treatment. And if surgery is not the best first step in your particular case (more on why this may be the case later), your surgeon will tell you this, explain why, and help get you set up with a medical oncologist.

It's worth spending some time thinking carefully about your choice of surgeon. A surgeon isn't just the person you are going to trust with your operation. A good breast surgeon will provide you with the critical information that you need to make the right decisions. In addition, he or she will get you set up with the right specialists that you may need to see for other parts of your treatment. For example, a plastic surgeon may be needed to participate in your surgery, and your breast surgeon would help you arrange that consultation. And as mentioned above, there are other specialists you may need to see after surgery is done. Depending on your case, a medical or radiation oncologist may need to be consulted for decision making regarding additional treatment (see chapters 9 and 10 on additional treatments that might be needed), and often your surgeon will help guide you toward the right specialists for those consultations as well.

Some women actually see a breast surgeon *before* they have been diagnosed with cancer, and this can be beneficial in many ways. While it may seem like overkill to consult a breast surgery specialist when you have to have a lump removed or a biopsy done and don't yet know if you have breast cancer, decision making regarding even the need for surgery and how it is performed can have a profound impact on your future care if a cancer is found, and it helps in terms of your confidence and continuity of care to know that you've started with the right person. Who is the right person? To start with, I highly recommend that you seek out a clinic or surgeon devoted to the treatment of breast cancer.

It may be that you look for or are referred to a general surgeon out of convenience simply to "get a diagnosis." My patient Melissa followed this course of action after she noticed a small knot in her upper right breast, near the armpit, about six months after her annual mammogram. The general surgeon who examined her—who had an office in the same building as Melissa's gynecologist, who recommended him—told her that he needed to take her to surgery to remove the lump right away, and that time was of the essence since it could be cancer. Melissa asked him whether it would be worthwhile to repeat the mammogram or conduct some other tests before rushing off to the operating room, but the surgeon said there was no reason for the mammogram to have changed, and that taking the lump out directly would be the best approach. Before she left the surgeon's office, Melissa scheduled the surgery for a few days later, but by the time she got home, she was feeling very uneasy about moving forward. She called my office, and I assured her that she was absolutely right to be concerned. She did *not* need to rush off to surgery, and there *were* other tests we could do to determine what was going on before racing to remove anything. What had originally seemed like a convenient decision to see a general surgeon ended up costing Melissa more time and stress in the long run.

Yes, it's true that general surgeons can perform breast surgery. In fact, breast surgery is taught as part of general surgery training, and so anyone who has been through a general surgery residency is qualified, at least on paper, to operate on a breast cancer patient. Up until the late 1970s and early 1980s, going to a general surgeon was the standard model of care for women with breast cancer. At that time, there was a limited amount that the surgeon needed to know about treating breast cancer, and only one operation: the radical mastectomy. No one spent any time or needed much specialized training to discuss the options, because there weren't any options to discuss!

In the modern era of breast cancer care, however, there is a much larger range of options and issues, most of which are quite complex: lumpectomy versus mastectomy, for example, or mastectomy versus bilateral mastectomy (for more on this, go to chapter 6). And that's even before we get to choices around sentinel lymph node biopsy, the management of lymph nodes, the role of genetics, and MRI and other imaging (discussed elsewhere in the book). A general surgeon performing an appendectomy on Monday, gall bladder surgery on Tuesday, and a breast cancer surgery on Wednesday cannot realistically be expected to have the knowledge base or expertise to guide you through all of the complex issues that are critical to making the right decisions for your care in the same way that a specialist working only on breast cancer cases every day of the week can.

Of course, patients may not have a wide variety of options when it comes to surgeons. Women who live in small towns or rural areas will most likely end up going to the one and only surgeon in their area who performs breast cancer surgery as part of his or her general surgical practice. If you don't have a qualified breast cancer specialist near you, however, you might want to consider traveling, if you can. Sometimes this may be impossible financially or because of logistical limitations or insurance constraints; the operating surgeon may be a matter of assignment rather than choice. But if *at all* possible, your priority at this early stage should be getting to a place where you will get the highest level of care, and that will be with a specialized breast cancer surgeon, known also as a breast surgical oncologist.

Choosing the right surgeon

If you are fortunate to have a choice of surgeons, you're most likely going to look to family and friends or to your physician for guidance. If someone you know and trust has had a good experience with her surgeon, it is worth pursuing that as a starting point. But do keep in mind that most laypeople do not have the ability to truly assess the skills and judgment of a surgeon, much less to have an understanding of what actually goes on in the operating room. Your neighbor's opinion of her surgeon is based mostly on subjective factors such as the surgeon's personality, the convenient location of his or her office, and the service and efficiency of the office staff. It's not that these factors aren't important—it's key to feel like you connect with the person who will be operating on you, and it could become important that you can get to the doctor's office without a long drive—but these factors should also be weighed against more critical ones.

If you do have a choice, here are the big three questions to ask:

1. **Is the surgeon dedicated to breast surgery as the mainstay of his or her practice?** There is just so much to know about breast cancer. And a huge part of being a breast surgery specialist is not just doing the actual operation, but rather the decision making that leads up to it. Thanks to exciting research, each year brings more advances and improvements in the standard of care for breast cancer surgery and treatment. Keeping up with the latest for breast cancer alone is challenging enough, and a surgeon who has to do this as well as stay up to date on other types of diseases and their management may not be able to offer the same level of expertise and focus.

2. **How many breast operations does the surgeon perform each week, month, or year?** There is clear-cut data demonstrating that surgeons and centers that do a high volume of specific types of surgery have better outcomes. This has been shown for various cancer types, including lung, prostate, and breast. It makes sense: a surgeon who performs more operations of the same type per month is better at the job than a surgeon who performs a range of surgeries in different categories, or only a few of one type. Usually with a breast specialist, high volume is a given.

   But finding someone who performs a high number of breast operations can be harder than it sounds. In New York State, data from as recently as 2002 show that approximately 75 percent of breast operations are performed by surgeons who do fewer than sixteen breast operations a year. It's highly unlikely that a surgeon performing one to two breast operations a month can have the same level of expertise, experience, and knowledge regarding appropriate management as someone who performs ten or more operations a week (as I and many of my breast surgery colleagues do). So look for that high volume.

3. **Has the surgeon completed a breast cancer fellowship?** Another way to identify excellence is to ask about your surgeon's level of qualification. For more than a decade now, advanced training in breast surgery has been offered as a one-year accredited fellowship. What this means is that surgeons who plan on devoting their careers to the treatment of patients with breast disease can spend an additional year beyond general surgical

training to focus on their area of interest. During this time, surgeons can gain an increased depth of understanding and learn the newest, most advanced techniques from the experts. There are top-notch fellowship positions all over the country devoted to training breast surgery specialists. A surgeon who has been through this type of fellowship is much more likely to have the knowledge base required to deliver the highest quality of care, and he or she has shown a commitment to breast surgery as a specialty. So if your surgeon has been in practice for less than ten years, it's worth asking if he or she did a breast surgery fellowship.

A WORD TO THE WISE

While friends and family can be a wonderful source of support and may be able to recommend good medical centers and doctors for your care, there's always the danger that their input can become overwhelming. As you begin the process of diagnosis and treatment, my advice is to be wary of people offering unsolicited advice: the websites you must read, the long email threads with words of caution from friends of friends of friends, the phone calls, the texts. While there is no doubt that most people are doing this from a place of kindness, it would be hard for these friends or family members to provide any meaningful information about your care without having knowledge of the specific details of your case. So don't let the onslaught of input upset your clarity and confuse your decision making during this crucial time.

The rest of the surgery team

Surgery is not the only aspect of your treatment, and so it follows that your surgeon is not the only person you will meet during your diagnosis and treatment. Your surgeon is part of a team, and the team is only as strong as its weakest link. You may have found a wonderful surgeon— someone who is kind and compassionate and who gave your friend the most beautiful incision in the world—but a surgeon cannot operate (literally or figuratively) in a vacuum. For example, in many cases, reconstruction is performed at the same time as the surgery for cancer, and thus a plastic surgeon will be involved. In such cases, the breast surgeon and plastic surgeon operate together, as a tag team: the breast surgeon goes first, and the plastic surgeon comes in afterward to reconstruct the removed breast. Because the breast and plastic surgeons must be able to work together, at the same facility or institution, usually the breast surgeon will refer you to a plastic surgeon with whom he or she works regularly.

In fact, the list of team members required for an excellent surgical result is quite extensive: anesthesiologists are critical, operating room nurses and technicians prepare the right equipment and make sure it is well serviced, technicians process the pathology specimens, pathologists examine the tissue removed, secretaries schedule the correct procedure. Everyone must be part of an integrated, specialized team.

When this doesn't happen, the quality of care may not be at its highest level. For example, if the surgeon performs a perfect operation but the hospital's pathologist does a less than perfect job examining the piece of tissue removed, then the surgeon's ability to make the right decisions and recommendations regarding your care will be compromised. In certain situations it can be hard for a pathologist who doesn't see a lot of breast cancer cases to distinguish between a cancer and something that is benign. Similarly, surgeons frequently depend on radiologists to localize an area before surgery so that it is easier to identify the tissue that needs to be removed. The surgeon's ability to retrieve the correct area is completely dependent on the radiologist's level of precision during the localization procedure (for more on this, see chapter 6).

In the best-case scenario, you would be able to go to a major medical or cancer center where breast cancer is treated regularly and in substantial volume. Excellent care may very well be available at the local surgicenter in town, but if not, don't feel that you have to settle. It will make a difference if you go elsewhere. As one of my former mentors used to say, "We may not cure everybody with good surgery, but we are not going to cure anybody without it."

The other specialists who may be required for subsequent parts of your treatment include a medical oncologist, who prescribes chemotherapy treatments and medicine, and a radiation oncologist, who gives radiation when necessary. Again, not all women need to see all of these specialists, and your surgeon should be able to guide you through the ensuing steps and get you connected to the doctors you need to see. The most common sequence for seeing these specialists is surgeon first, medical oncologist second, and radiation oncologist third. Under some circumstances, your surgeon may want you to see a medical oncologist *before* surgery is performed, and chemotherapy may even be recommended prior to surgery (for more on chemotherapy before surgery, see chapter 9). If this is a possible course of treatment, your surgeon and medical oncologist should work together with you to devise the best plan for your care.

Putting together your team: "all under one roof" versus "mix and match" from different places

You and your doctors should work together to make sure your care flows seamlessly from one phase to the next. One way to do this is to have your care in a specialized breast cancer center, where all aspects of care are given under one roof. Doctors who work together regularly as a team in a high-volume center, especially within a recognized medical center, can often provide the highest level of care. In the Dubin Breast Center at Mount Sinai Hospital, where I work, we have all of the specialists one might need for any aspect of breast cancer diagnosis or treatment working adjacent to each other and available within one facility. Within a specialized center such as this, surgeons can review their patients' films side by side with radiologists to optimize plans for care. Patients who discover a new lump on a routine follow-up exam with one of their doctors can be taken immediately to radiology, down the hall, for further imaging and evaluation without delay. If any lab or imaging tests are done, all doctors have access to the results. And when difficult or complicated cases arise, doctors of all disciplines convene in "tumor board" meetings, putting their heads together to come up with the best plan. From a practical standpoint, specialized centers often enable doctors to arrange expeditious appointments for their patients with the other doctors, allowing patients to easily move through the system. In most major medical centers and their breast centers, doctors also share centralized electronic medical records, which means that you don't have to worry about making sure information is transmitted from one doctor to the next, or about critical details slipping through the cracks.

Many women, however, choose to mix and match, having different aspects of their care in different places. I have many patients who come from all over to New York City to have me perform their surgery but then prefer to stay closer to home for other parts of their care, which involve more frequent visits or treatment that would be inconvenient to travel for. You may find that after seeking different opinions you like one doctor at one medical center for surgery but another in a private practice office for medical oncology. While this arrangement may require you to take more initiative in order to keep all your doctors on the same page and make sure records are transmitted back and forth, seamless care can still be easily accomplished with different doctors' offices faxing and emailing, which is done all the time.

When a second opinion is needed

Sometimes it may be necessary to seek a second opinion. Examples of when I think you should consider getting one have already been pointed out in previous chapters, and I will continue to point out other instances when getting a second opinion may be warranted. But they are not always necessary. Second opinions are an option but not an obligation. If the surgeon you have already seen meets all the requirements discussed above, there is really no reason you *must* get a second opinion.

In my practice, I often see patients whose friends and family members are pushing for second opinions because they feel that "this is what you are supposed to do." Although these friends and family members are well-meaning, their advice can sometimes be misguided.

To give you an example: After a needle biopsy, Jill, a forty-three-year-old mother of two, learned she had two small cancers in separate areas of her right breast. I met with Jill to discuss the options, and we decided together that mastectomy—removing the whole breast with the cancer—was the best choice for her. With her husband and her closest friend at the appointment, we discussed the approach at length and proceeded to schedule surgery. A few days later Jill called to say she was receiving a lot of pressure from another friend to see a surgeon at a different hospital for a second opinion. This friend, Sarah, had had a double mastectomy with the same surgeon earlier in the year.

Jill and I had a long, frank discussion. I said I had absolutely no problem with her seeing another doctor for a second opinion, and Jill certainly had time to do so, as her scheduled surgery was approximately two weeks away. I also told her that I was completely confident that the plan we had chosen together was the right one and that there was no reason in her particular case to remove the other, healthy breast. Jill did go to see the other doctor, who made the same recommendation as I had, and ultimately we proceeded with surgery as planned. During one of our follow-up visits, Jill indicated to me that she felt as though her friend was strongly advocating for her to have a double mastectomy, as that was what had worked for her. But no two cancer cases are the same, and it's important that you make your decision in collaboration with your surgeon and on your own terms.

That said, there's no doubt that a second opinion can often be quite reassuring, as it was for Jill. Sometimes you are just so overwhelmed at the first appointment that hearing it all again from another doctor, in perhaps a slightly different way, is exactly what you need. Even if the second doctor says the same thing as the first, often it all seems to make more sense the second time around. I call this the "repetition factor." It's all so new, you may simply need to hear it more than once. And of course a second opinion becomes especially important if you harbor any doubts about the path you have chosen or the place you have chosen for your care. If your surgeon or facility does not meet the standards outlined above, then I would say a second opinion is probably an excellent idea. A good second opinion facility will ask you to bring in all the materials leading up to your diagnosis, including your radiology pictures and your pathology slides (which show the tissue that was removed at the time of biopsy). They'll also take into account your personal and family history, and based on all these factors, you'll receive a completely independent review, assessment, and recommendation.

If you do decide to seek a second opinion, it's important that you don't sit in the second doctor's office explaining in detail the first doctor's recommendation. When I hear patients launching into a lengthy description of the other doctor's plan, I usually cut them off, asking them to forgive my rudeness for interrupting. Then I explain that they are entitled to a completely unbiased second opinion and that this cannot happen if I first hear what the other doctor recommended. Once the patient has heard my recommendation, then we can talk about any discrepancies in the two opinions.

The first two opinions are different. Do you get a third opinion? Or a fourth? When should the information seeking end?

Sometimes when you reach the point of the third or fourth opinion, it becomes counterproductive to seek another opinion, only serving to delay decision making and getting the needed care. There are many women who understandably will never feel "ready" for surgery, but delaying treatment beyond more than a month or so can be detrimental. Most cases are straightforward enough that there shouldn't be that much difference of opinion about the important aspects of treatment. So if you find yourself in this position, make sure at least one of the opinions is from a top-notch center where you can have a high degree of confidence that their recommendations are reliable. Decide where you are most comfortable, and then move forward.

Getting the best care with limited financial resources and/or no health insurance at all

If you are already facing financial challenges, there's no doubt that a breast cancer diagnosis can be particularly devastating. It's hard enough managing your health needs without factoring in holding down a job or sometimes two, finding child care, and keeping up with your household responsibilities. For women in this situation, I highly recommend that you try to go to a major medical center if you can. Many of these centers have clinics that provide access to extensive resources such as social workers, financial planners, and organized and free support groups. These ancillary services can be critical sources of information and support to you and your family before, during, and after treatment.

For the significant number of women who do not have any health insurance, there are still options for solid, good care. Most major city and county medical centers across the country have clinics where young breast cancer specialists of all disciplines are working. There will most likely not be the same level of continuity of care as one would have with a private doctor, but receiving high-level care is still possible.

THE TAKEAWAY

- Find a breast surgery specialist who treats a large volume of patients and is well trained.
- The surgeon is part of a team, and a good center usually comes with a good team.

CHAPTER 5

Understanding Your Diagnosis

what you have and what it really means

Janet is a fifty-year-old attorney who came to my office after her biopsy showed a small area of invasive ductal cancer. She arrived with her biopsy pathology report in hand. From my side of the desk I could see that Janet had already highlighted, underlined, and annotated her copy of the report (like I used to do with my medical school textbooks) in an attempt to decipher the information on the page and assess its importance. I explained to Janet that at this early juncture, only a few key pieces of information provided by the report from the biopsy were actually useful and important in terms of her prognosis or guiding decisions about the next steps of treatment. We proceeded to go through these one by one. More information would come later, in the more lengthy pathology report from her surgery.

In the event that you *do* receive a breast cancer diagnosis, you're going to be introduced to all kinds of words and phrases, and it's understandable that it may take you a while to understand them and their significance. In this chapter, I'll provide you with a glossary of definitions to help you navigate your diagnosis and subsequent treatment.

What *is* breast cancer?

Breast cancer starts out as one cell in the breast that accumulates enough damage or change in its DNA that it loses normal control mechanisms and starts growing and dividing abnormally. Causes of this damage can be environmental, hereditary, or a combination of the two. When this one abnormal cell starts growing and dividing, it becomes two cells, then four cells, then eight, then . . . you get the picture. By the time this small mass of cancer cells reaches one centimeter, or a little less than half an inch, it already contains about one billion cells. And that's how cancer starts and develops. Other words you may hear to describe a cancer include "malignancy" and "tumor." In order to remove the cancer, surgery will need to be performed, possibly followed by additional treatment, depending on your type of cancer or surgery (for more on postsurgery treatments, go to chapters 9 and 10). In some instances, other types of treatment precede surgery (see the section on neoadjuvant chemotherapy in chapter 9).

When your surgeon speaks to you about your diagnosis, you're going to hear him or her speaking about the breast duct or the lobule. The lobule is where milk is made in the breast, and cancer that develops from here is called *lobular cancer.* The ducts are the milk delivery system, a pipelike network of tubes within the breast that all converge on the nipple. Cancer that develops within the duct is called *ductal cancer,* and is the most common type of breast cancer.

Types of breast cancer

DCIS or noninvasive cancer

Noninvasive cancer is also called *DCIS,* which stands for *ductal carcinoma in situ.* This is the earliest stage of breast cancer, which is why it's also known as stage 0 breast cancer. DCIS is most commonly detected by a mammogram, and it is usually—but not always—detected when it is still microscopic, before you might feel anything even close to a lump. (Occasionally DCIS will be detected by a new lump or possibly by bloody nipple discharge.) The "in situ" part of the name means "in its place," and with DCIS the cancer cells are contained within the duct of the breast, confined by the duct wall. With this type of cancer, the cancer cells are very unlikely to spread, since the superhighways for spread (the blood vessels and the lymphatic channels) exist *outside* the duct wall. If the cancer has not broken through the duct wall, then cancer cells have no on-ramp to the superhighway and therefore have a low likelihood of spread. Thanks to widespread mammographic screening, DCIS accounts for approximately 20 to 25 percent of all newly diagnosed breast cancer. And here's a real reason for optimism: if you are diagnosed with DCIS, the cure rate is approximately 98 to 99 percent. There are very few cancers, breast or otherwise, that are associated with such high cure rates.

Invasive or infiltrating cancers: invasive ductal cancer and invasive lobular cancer

If DCIS makes up approximately 20 to 25 percent of all cancers, invasive cancer is more common, making up the remaining 75 to 80 percent of all newly diagnosed cases of breast cancer. With an invasive cancer, also called infiltrating cancer, the cancer cells have broken through the duct wall. In these cases, the amount of cancer outside the duct is quantified by the size of the tumor, and the bigger the tumor, the higher the likelihood of spread. But it's important to know that even with invasive cancers, most that are diagnosed are small and have not spread, leading to the high rates of cure that we see today.

When breast cancer does spread, one of the first stops is the lymph nodes or glands under the arm. Unlike DCIS, where there is little potential for spread, with invasive cancer it's very important to check the lymph nodes, as there can be the potential for spread.

There are various types of invasive cancer. The most common kind originates in the milk ducts of the breast and is called *invasive* or *infiltrating ductal cancer* (accounting for approximately 80 percent of all invasive cancers). The second most common type of invasive breast cancer is called *invasive* or *infiltrating lobular cancer* because it originates in the lobules of the breast, where milk is made (this accounts for 10 percent of all invasive cancers). Invasive ductal and lobular cancers are treated essentially the same way and are associated with the same prognosis overall. Lobular cancers can be trickier to detect and have the reputation of being invisible on mammograms, growing more like sheets of cells and less like a discreet lump, and thus tend to be larger at the time of diagnosis.

Other, rarer cancers

DCIS, invasive ductal cancer, and invasive lobular cancer make up the vast majority of newly diagnosed breast cancer cases (approximately 95 percent). The last 5 to 10 percent of cancers are rare types, and include some cancers that are associated with a better prognosis and others that are associated with a worse prognosis. *Mucinous cancers* are rare and usually associated with smaller tumor size, lower likelihood of lymph node spread, and overall better prognosis. The same is true for *tubular cancers* and some *medullary cancers,* as well as *adenoid cystic cancers.*

On the other end of the spectrum, *inflammatory breast cancer,* which accounts for less than 1 percent of all new cancers, is an aggressive form of breast cancer that requires us to be even more aggressive in treating it. *Inflammatory breast cancer* is a type of breast cancer that involves not only the whole breast but usually the overlying skin as well. Inflammatory breast cancer can look like a skin rash or infection over an enlarged, swollen breast. The skin can also look thickened or pitted, giving it the characteristic appearance of an orange peel (doctors use the French term for this, *peau d'orange*). Making the diagnosis of inflammatory breast cancer can sometimes be dangerously delayed when the patient is presumed to have an infection and is treated with antibiotics for a prolonged period of time, without improvement. Ultimately, a physician does a breast biopsy and sometimes a biopsy of the affected overlying breast skin to finally make the diagnosis. (See chapter 6 for more on the specifics of treatment of this type of cancer.)

Paget's disease is an uncommon kind of breast cancer that involves the nipple, either exclusively or with the underlying breast. Paget's disease is often detected as visible changes to the nipple, and some patients are referred to a dermatologist first when they complain of a rash or scabbing specifically of the nipple. A nipple biopsy can often make the diagnosis of Paget's disease.

In *occult breast cancer,* which accounts for 1 percent of new breast cancer cases, the first abnormality that is identified is a mass in the armpit (a lymph node with cancer) even while the breast exam and mammogram are normal. A cancerous lymph node in the armpit could be a sign of some other cancer, such as lymphoma or melanoma. In most cases in women, however, the lymph node will be related to an occult or hidden cancer within the breast that is just too small to detect but aggressive enough to have already started to spread.

For more on these rare cancers and their treatment models, go to chapter 6.

SURGICAL TERMINOLOGY

For most cases of newly diagnosed breast cancer, both DCIS and invasive, the first step in treatment is surgery, either lumpectomy or mastectomy, with lymph node assessment in cases of invasive breast cancer and some cases of DCIS (see below for more on lymph nodes).

Lumpectomy

There are many different names for lumpectomy: *wide excision, breast conservation, limited resection, quadrantectomy,* even *partial mastectomy.* All of these names refer to essentially the same procedure, which involves making a small incision in the breast and taking out an area of tissue, including the cancer, while leaving most of the breast intact. In the majority of cases, lumpectomy is followed by radiation treatment.

Lumpectomy is one of the most significant advances in the history of breast cancer treatment. Until the 1970s and early 1980s the only operation that was effective for curing breast cancer was radical mastectomy, a dramatic, disfiguring operation that involved removing not only the entire breast but also the underlying pectoralis muscle, leaving a severe depression in the chest wall that could not be reconstructed. Remember, back then women did not routinely get mammograms, or any other breast cancer screening test for that matter, so by the time the cancer was diagnosed, it usually had grown to a sizable mass and could not be removed effectively with anything other than this extensive operation.

In the 1980s, as the use of mammography increased and imaging technology improved, we could begin to detect smaller and smaller cancers. Landmark trials were performed in the United States, Italy, and other countries comparing mastectomy with the lumpectomy, a more limited operation where only part of the breast is removed. When lumpectomy was followed by radiation, the outcomes were comparable to those seen for mastectomy: a low risk of recurrence in the breast and *absolutely equivalent survival rates*. As a result of this proven equivalence, most women diagnosed with early breast cancer—whether DCIS or invasive—now have *two* viable and equally effective options for their surgical treatment: lumpectomy plus radiation or mastectomy. Most women who are diagnosed with breast cancer are eligible for lumpectomy, and most women who are eligible for lumpectomy choose this option. Keep in mind that breast cancer is really the only disease where doctors can offer two very different options for surgery with equivalent outcomes, thereby offering most patients a choice.

Mastectomy

Mastectomy is the second option for breast cancer surgery. Like lumpectomy, it is performed for women with both DCIS and invasive cancer, and sometimes to prevent breast cancer for women at very high risk for developing breast cancer (see chapter 15 for more on women who are at very high risk). Most women who receive a mastectomy also opt for breast reconstruction (for more on mastectomy and reconstruction techniques, go to chapters 6 and 7). When you choose to have reconstruction, the first stage is usually performed at the same time as mastectomy, so you wake up from surgery with some semblance of a breast shape. There may be additional steps and smaller procedures to complete the reconstruction process a few months later, after you have recovered from the first, larger procedure. When no reconstruction is performed, modern-day mastectomy techniques do not remove the pec muscle, so the chest wall is flat after surgery but not concave, as it used to be after a radical mastectomy performed in the old days. When both breasts are removed we call this a bilateral mastectomy, also referred to as a double mastectomy.

Lymph nodes

Lymph nodes or glands are small round masses of tissue that can be found throughout the body but tend to congregate in certain areas we call lymph node basins. Lymph node basins can be found on both sides of the neck, above and below the collarbone or clavicle, under the arms, throughout the chest and belly, and in the groin. Normal lymph nodes can vary in size from the head of a pin to a grape; most are about the shape and size of a lima bean. Women have lots of lymph nodes under the arm, anywhere from ten to fifty.

Nodes are filled with cells from the immune system, and these cells travel in fluid called lymph that flows through a network of vessels called lymphatics. This complex system—the lymphatic system—functions as a kind of filtration system for the body, with the lymph nodes serving as the bunkers for the lymphatic system and its cells. These nodes can get swollen for many reasons, but mostly they do so as a reaction to infection or trauma, as they are packed with cells for fighting infection. For example, when you have a sore throat, your body fights the infection by sending tons of cellular reinforcements to the neighboring lymph nodes so they can launch their attack against the invading infection. This explains why, when you have that sore throat, you may develop a swollen gland or node in the neck: your body is actually arming itself for fighting off the infection.

Lymph nodes can also be the first line of defense against the spread of cancer. When breast cancer starts to spread, usually its first stop is the lymph nodes under the arm on the side of the cancer, also called *axillary nodes*. When cancer has started to spread to the lymph nodes and the spread is still microscopic, there is usually nothing that one can feel on examination or see with the naked eye to determine that this has happened. As a result, if we want to find out if cancer has spread to the nodes, we usually have to remove one or more of them so we can look at them under the microscope (see the section on sentinel lymph node biopsy, below, for information on how we know what to look for). When there has been a substantial amount of spread of cancer cells and the nodes are filled with them, one can often feel or see that the nodes are enlarged or firm. In advanced cases, breast cancer can also spread regionally to other lymph node groups, including the internal mammary nodes, which are inside the sternum (breastbone), and the supraclavicular nodes, which are above the clavicle (collarbone). Spread to these areas is not common. Lymph nodes in the neck can be checked for obvious spread by physical examination. Internal mammary nodes cannot be assessed by physical examination since they live inside the chest, but they can be seen on scans of the body, which are done in advanced cases. So for most women, checking lymph nodes for spread focuses on the axillary lymph nodes, under the arm on the same side of the body as the tumor.

For women with DCIS who are having a lumpectomy, in most cases checking lymph nodes is not routinely recommended as part of surgery, given the extremely low likelihood of spread. For women with invasive cancer, however, checking lymph nodes to find out if cancer has spread is routine in almost all cases. The likelihood of lymph node spread increases directly in relation to tumor size. If you have a one-centimeter cancer, you have about a 10 percent chance of node spread. If you have a two-centimeter cancer, you have a 20 percent chance of node spread. (These are approximations and there are other factors involved, but in general they provide a crude estimate of risk.)

For women with invasive breast cancer, it's important to find out the true status of the lymph nodes for two main reasons:

1. If there is a significant amount of cancer in the lymph nodes, we want to remove it along with the cancer in the breast. It makes no sense to take such great care to remove cancer in the breast while leaving it behind someplace else.
2. Lymph node involvement and the number of nodes involved is one of the most important factors in determining cancer stage, prognosis, and whether additional treatments such as chemotherapy are needed.

Axillary dissection

Before the mid-1990s, all lymph nodes were checked the same way—we had to remove all the nodes so we could examine them individually under the microscope. This operation is called an *axillary dissection*. The problem with axillary dissection is that because it involves removing all the nodes, it's fairly extensive surgery. As a result, it's associated with side effects such as swelling in the arm, numbness, and an increased risk of infection for the arm or breast on the side where the surgery was performed.

It's important to know that when we do have to remove most or all of the nodes from under the arm, this does not affect your body's overall immune system. There are thousands of other nodes left in other basins in the body, and so this should not be a concern for any woman. Also important to know is that when cancer spreads to nodes under one arm, it doesn't mean nodes under the other arm need to be checked. Thankfully, cancer rarely jumps from one side of the body to the other. When you have an axillary dissection, we usually leave a drain. A drain is a rubber tube with small perforations that is threaded through a small hole in the skin and sits under the arm in the space that the lymph nodes formerly occupied. The drain collects the lymph fluid that the nodes normally filter. Over the days and weeks following surgery, as the body heals, the fluid becomes reabsorbed through other pathways, and drainage tapers off; eventually the drain is removed in the doctor's office. (For more on axillary dissection recovery, see chapter 12.)

Sentinel node biopsy

In the mid-1990s, pioneering surgeons decided to figure out if there was a way to check the status of the lymph nodes without having to remove them all, thereby avoiding the larger axillary dissection and its associated potential long-term risks. The procedure that was developed to accomplish this goal is called *sentinel lymph node biopsy*. The basic premise of sentinel node biopsy is that in any given grouping of lymph nodes, there are one or more gatekeeper or "sentinel" nodes. If the cancer is going to spread, it would go directly to the sentinel nodes before spreading to the other nodes. Sentinel node biopsy identifies those key gatekeeper nodes so that they can be cherry-picked out from the larger group and examined under the microscope. If the sentinel nodes are normal, we can conclude that the cancer has not taken the first step to spread and the rest of the lymph nodes are normal too. We can then feel comfortable leaving the rest of the lymph nodes in place, and a much smaller operation has been performed, with much less risk of developing the complications associated with axillary dissection. Alternatively, if the nodes are abnormal, the surgeon can then proceed to do an axillary dissection if needed, especially if there is a strong possibility of more cancer in the rest of the nodes.

Sentinel lymph node biopsy is now the standard of care for evaluating the lymph nodes under the arm. In order to figure out which node or nodes are the sentinel nodes, we use liquid dye, injecting it into the breast immediately before surgery. The dye then travels through the breast tissue via the lymphatic pathways to a select node or few nodes under the arm. Keep in mind that the path of the dye does not tell us if the cancer has spread; it tells us where the cancer would go first if it *did* spread. In many cases the dye goes to more than one lymph node; often two or three light up with the dye and need to be removed and checked. Depending on the type of surgery and the institution, sometimes lymph nodes will be sent to the laboratory during surgery, while the patient is still asleep on the table. A quick test, known as a frozen section or touch prep, is conducted to see if there is any obvious cancer there. The benefit of these tests is that if cancer is seen, the results can be communicated to the surgeon in the operating room, and if an axillary dissection is needed, it can be performed during the same operation. In other circumstances, sentinel nodes are removed and sent to the lab for analysis in the days after surgery. If nodes prove positive on later analysis, sometimes a second operation is required to remove the remaining nodes.

With invasive cancer, an evaluation of the lymph nodes under the arm should be performed in almost all cases; this information is critical to determining cancer stage and weighs heavily in decision making about the need for additional treatments. Sentinel node biopsy can usually be omitted in cases of DCIS being treated with lumpectomy. (In the small chance that invasive cancer is found, we can always go back and inject dye into the remaining breast, which would accurately show us which nodes need to be removed in a second operation.)

NEED TO KNOW

With DCIS, sentinel node biopsy should always be performed for patients who need or choose to have a mastectomy. In these cases, a sentinel node biopsy is performed at the same time as the surgery. It's important to do this because occasionally invasive cancer will be unexpectedly found in the mastectomy tissue, and if the surgery is already done, we can't go back and perform sentinel node biopsy because there is no way to inject dye into the breast (a necessary part of sentinel node biopsy) once that breast has been removed.

Sentinel node biopsy has been around now for approximately twenty years, and there have been multiple, reputable trials demonstrating the effectiveness and accuracy of the procedure. It is now considered an integral part of the standard of care. If your surgeon does not perform sentinel node biopsy or voices concern regarding the reliability of the procedure, then you can know with certainty that your surgeon is someone who is *not* up to speed with current standards of practice for breast cancer (or who performs so little breast surgery that he or she has not mastered the technique). In other words, if you have invasive breast cancer where lymph nodes are not known to be involved and need to be checked, and your surgeon does not plan on performing sentinel lymph node biopsy, you really need to find another surgeon.

Although we now use sentinel node biopsy to identify and remove individual nodes, eliminating the need for axillary dissection in most cases, there are still situations in which axillary dissection needs to be performed, and where the sentinel lymph node biopsy is *not* necessary or should not be performed:

1. Sometimes before the surgery, the surgeon actually feels suspicious lymph nodes under the arm on physical examination or the radiologist sees suspicious lymph nodes on a mammogram or sonogram. When this happens, a small needle biopsy can be performed to sample the suspicious node or nodes before any surgery is done. If the results come back a day or two later confirming cancer involving the lymph nodes, there is usually no reason to check further with a sentinel node biopsy at the time of surgery. Instead, the surgeon can simply proceed to performing an axillary dissection. If the lymph nodes are found to be positive prior to surgery, indicating the cancer has taken the first step toward spreading, scans of the body may be recommended to provide better information about the possible further extent of cancer spread.

2. Another situation where sentinel lymph node biopsy is not necessary is when patients have very advanced cancer—for example, inflammatory breast cancer (see chapters 5 and 6). If the surgeon knows that the risk of lymph node involvement is so high that it is almost certain, sometimes sentinel node biopsy to check the nodes is bypassed and the surgeon proceeds right to axillary dissection; however, these cases are rare.

Lymphedema

Lymphedema is the main long-term risk or side effect of performing an axillary dissection. Lymph nodes are part of the body's filtration system, and lymph is the fluid that circulates around the body, carrying cells from the immune system to fight sources of infection. When lymph nodes under the arm are removed and lymphatic pathways are cut, it's possible for fluid to accumulate in the arm. In this scenario, the swelling is called lymphedema ("edema" means swelling), and this can also be associated with numbness and increased risk of infection in the arm.

The risk of lymphedema after an axillary dissection is approximately 20 percent, but it can be higher in women who are obese and in those who also require radiation directed at the nodes after surgery (see chapter 10 for more information on when radiation is needed after lymph node surgery). Symptoms of lymphedema vary enormously. They can be mild, making a woman feel just a little puffy (almost like she would feel after eating a meal that was too salty, but just in one arm). Less frequently, symptoms can be severe, and these are the pictures you will see if you Google lymphedema. My advice is to avoid looking at these images, as it is rare for cases to be this exaggerated. Symptoms can be chronic and unremitting, or they can come and go, brought on by certain activities and then subsiding.

NEED TO KNOW

There is also a small risk of developing lymphedema if you have only a sentinel lymph node biopsy, but the risk is much, much lower—approximately 2 percent—and it's why sentinel node biopsy represents such an advance over axillary dissection for women with normal lymph nodes.

There are various dos and don'ts aimed at reducing the risk of lymphedema after having an axillary dissection. The don'ts include the taking of blood pressure (due to the squeezing and constriction of the arm), getting blood drawn from that arm, or any other activities that can expose the hand or arm to increased risk of infection (including gardening without a glove or getting a manicure and trimming the cuticles too closely). The dos include a range of strengthening and range-of-motion exercises, starting after surgery and building over time. Although we used to tell patients that early exercise might increase the risk of lymphedema, we now believe the opposite is true. Early mobilization may actually reduce the risk of lymphedema by healing and rebuilding remaining lymphatic pathways. Your breast surgeon will be able to talk to you about the possibility of developing lymphedema and what you can do to mitigate the risks. Many will also refer patients to physical therapists who are familiar with techniques to reduce the risk, and that is fine too.

THE TAKEAWAY

- DCIS is noninvasive cancer. About 20 to 25 percent of newly diagnosed breast cancer falls into this category, and cure rates are as high as 99 percent.
- The two most common types of invasive cancer are invasive ductal cancer and invasive lobular cancer.
- Checking lymph nodes for cancer spread is important for almost all women with invasive cancer, as well as some with DCIS, and is achieved with sentinel node biopsy.
- Axillary dissection, removing most or all of the lymph nodes under the arm, is reserved for those with known and extensive lymph node spread.

CHAPTER 6

One of the Biggest Decisions

lumpectomy versus mastectomy

After my patient Laura was diagnosed with breast cancer, she came into my office for a consultation. She had been referred by two of her closest friends, women whom I had also treated. When we discussed Laura's options, lumpectomy and mastectomy, Laura was surprised to learn that I thought lumpectomy with radiation to follow was a perfectly appropriate choice for her. Both of her friends had had mastectomies, and one of them had had both breasts removed (bilateral mastectomy). Laura assumed that would be my recommendation for her too.

I told Laura what I tell all my patients, and what's become a central message in this book as well: when it comes to making decisions about breast cancer surgery, one size definitely does not fit all. There are many variables, and each of these variables can mean something different for each individual woman. As surgeons, we need to take into account so many factors, including age, overall health, breast size, cancer size, family history, and, last and most important, *what does the patient want?* Decision making regarding breast cancer surgery is both medical *and* personal, and even two people who seem like they have exactly the same case may end up with two very different recommendations and outcomes.

Breast cancer is one of the only diseases where, in the majority of cases, patients actually have a choice about what kind of surgery they will receive. There is really no other tumor type where the surgeon and patient collaborate on deciding about the extent of the surgery. A colon surgeon doesn't usually say to a patient, "Listen, do you want me to remove fifteen centimeters of your colon or twenty?" The lung cancer surgeon doesn't ask, "Do you want me to take a big piece of your left lung or a small piece?" And even if these surgeons did ask you to choose, those differences wouldn't be noticeable from the outside. However, for most women, the decision to remove the whole breast or just part of it is a highly charged decision that measurably impacts the way she looks and feels.

Not everyone will have a choice. In some cases, mastectomy is clearly the better way to go; in others, lumpectomy is obviously preferable. But for the majority of patients, there is a range of options. Should you have a small surgery with radiation or a bigger surgery alone? Should you remove the other breast? Reconstruction or no reconstruction? Implant or tissue reconstruction?

During the decision-making process, you want to make sure you have all the bases covered, and that you are making a well-informed decision. Sometimes the difficulty involved in making this decision and the need to make the "right" decision drive information seeking. When information comes from a doctor who knows the details of your case, this can bring clarity and empower you to make the best decision. When information comes from people in your wider circle or online sources, it can often have the opposite effect. What I've seen from treating thousands of patients in my years as a breast surgeon is that the best way to deal with the decision-making process is to stay calm, know that you have some time, and be ready to tune out the background noise. With the right guidance, you will truly come to the right decision for *you*.

Lumpectomy: how it's done

With lumpectomy, the surgeon makes a small incision in the breast and removes an area of tissue that contains the cancer. Sometimes the surgeon will take additional pieces of surrounding tissue to increase the chances that the cancer has been completely removed. The wound is then closed, usually with dissolvable stitches, and the body then naturally fills in the empty cavity in the breast with fluid, blood, and ultimately scar tissue.

Every patient undergoing lumpectomy wants to know how much tissue will be removed and what the breast will look like after surgery. In general, the amount of tissue removed is directly related to the size of the actual cancer, since the cancer needs to be removed in its entirety until there are clear margins (edges) all the way around. Although everyone heals differently, with a well-performed lumpectomy the size and shape of the breast should not change very much (unless the tumor is very large and/or your breast is very small) and the scar should fade over time.

Localization

In many breast cancer cases, you and your surgeon can actually feel the cancerous lump manually, and so the incision is simply made on or near where the lump is felt. But in most cases, thanks to screening and early detection, the cancer may be so small that it cannot be seen or felt without the help and guidance of a mammogram or other imaging test; it may even be microscopic. So how does a surgeon find the area of cancer if it cannot be felt or seen with the naked eye? In these cases, surgeons use a *localization procedure* done prior to surgery to localize the right area.

Localization can be done two different ways:

1. *Wire localization* is the most common and widely used method. With wire localization, you undergo an imaging study, usually a mammogram or ultrasound, right before the surgery. During that test, the area of the cancer is identified (remember the critical clip to mark the spot in chapter 2?), some local anesthesia is injected into the breast skin, and a skinny wire is advanced into the breast to the target. The wire has a small hook on the end so that it wedges into the tissue and won't slip out or become dislodged. The other end of the wire protrudes through the skin and is taped down well and secured. You are then escorted to the

operating room with the wire in place. Once you are in the operating room and deeper anesthesia is administered, the surgeon makes a cut near where the wire is protruding, follows the wire down like a guidepost to its end and removes the surrounding area corresponding to the cancer. Frequently the surgeon will take an X-ray or mini-mammogram of the area of tissue that was removed (the lumpectomy specimen). Most operating rooms where large numbers of breast procedures are performed have these special X-ray machines in or near the operating room suites to do this expeditiously. The X-ray can show the surgeon in real time that he or she has successfully retrieved the correct area by showing that the cancer (or the metal clip left in at the time of biopsy to mark the spot corresponding to the cancer) is present in the area of tissue removed. It is important to note that wire or needle localization can only be performed immediately before the surgery, as you cannot walk around for days with a wire hanging out of your breast!

2. *Seed localization* is a newer procedure. With seed localization, a tiny radioactive chip, the size of a small staple, is deposited into the breast through a skinny needle in order to mark the spot. The radioactive seed gives off a signal that can be detected by a special probe that we have in the operating room. While wire localization should really only be done the morning of surgery, seed localization has the distinct advantage of being able to be done days or weeks before the surgery. Because the seed is implanted within the breast, there is no real risk of dislodgement, and the signal persists, unheard and undetected, until you arrive in the operating room. Once you are asleep, we use the probe to lead us to the seed signal. We can then make our incision on the surface of the breast directly overlying the signal and follow it down to the target. As with wire localization, we can take an X-ray to verify that our tiny target has been retrieved. As seed localization does not have to be done on the actual day of surgery, it potentially reduces the associated anxiety and discomfort that can prevail on a long day of surgery when wire localization is performed.

A WORD TO THE WISE

If you are having a lumpectomy, there are two technical aspects of the procedure that you should discuss with your surgeon before your operation: the incision and the orientation of the cancer specimen that is removed. Unfortunately, some surgeons who are not breast specialists fail to consider these two key factors when performing their operations.

1. If at all possible, the incision should be made in the same direction as the skin's natural lines (the subtle gradations on the surface of the breast). Surgeons who are breast specialists are trained to do this and are aware of this principle going into every operation. So while it would be a bad idea to demand that the surgeon tell you exactly where and how big the incision will be, my advice is that you ask your surgeon to describe the *approximate* location and orientation of the incision that will be made. In the unlikely eventuality that you need a mastectomy after your lumpectomy—because more cancer has been found than was initially estimated—an incision made along the breast's natural lines will minimize the total amount of skin that needs to be removed during the second surgery.

2. The orientation of the cancer specimen is equally important. When the piece of tissue with the cancer is removed, it's generally in the shape of a sphere. In order to orient the specimen, your surgeon carefully marks the piece of tissue in a way that tells the pathologist which edges of the specimen correspond to which part of the body. If it turns out that more surgery is needed, then a clear picture of the orientation will minimize the amount of tissue that needs to be removed in the next operation. Let's say one of the edges of the sphere is shown to be "positive." Your surgeon can then go back to the cavity and selectively remove more tissue in the problematic area. If the specimen is not oriented, then your surgeon has no ability to determine which part of the specimen corresponds to which edge in the breast. This means he or she has to go back and remove *all* the edges all the way around, a process involving taking out more tissue than was otherwise necessary, which can leave greater indentation and disfigurement.

Mastectomy: how it's done

In essence, a standard mastectomy operation involves making an incision above and below the nipple, separating skin away from underlying breast tissue, and removing *all* of the breast tissue along with the overlying nipple and some surrounding skin. This is done under general anesthesia.

There are many different subtypes of mastectomies. The ancestor of mastectomies is the radical mastectomy, an extremely extensive and disfiguring operation that is rarely performed anymore. Once mammography was introduced and tumors were found at earlier stages and when they were smaller, a more limited version of the mastectomy was adopted.

When a woman with breast cancer needs or chooses to have a mastectomy, one of the most important parts of the breast surgeon's job is to figure out which type of mastectomy should be performed to maximize chances of a good cosmetic outcome without risking leaving cancer behind.

Here are the various types of mastectomy surgery that are currently standard:

1. The *modified radical mastectomy* removes the breast, including the nipple, and the lymph nodes, but preserves the pectoralis muscle. While modified radical mastectomy is still disfiguring, it is slightly less so than the radical mastectomy, as the pec muscle is preserved, leaving a flat chest wall rather than a concave one. This procedure is the standard for tumors that are large and have spread to the lymph nodes but don't invade the underlying pec muscle.

2. The *total mastectomy* or *simple mastectomy* is the same as the modified radical mastectomy (even though the names sound very different) in that it involves removing all the breast tissue and the nipple and preserving the pec muscle. The main difference between the modified radical mastectomy and the total mastectomy is simply the extent of lymph node removal (and the terminology isn't intuitive): with the modified radical, all of the lymph nodes are removed, while with the total mastectomy, most of the lymph nodes are actually preserved.

3. The *skin-sparing mastectomy* is essentially the same as a total or simple mastectomy where we remove the nipple, but save the majority of the surrounding skin envelope. This surgery can only be performed with simultaneous breast reconstruction.

4. The *nipple-sparing mastectomy* preserves the nipple and surrounding areola but still removes all of the underlying breast tissue and the breast ducts that go up into the nipple. Again, this can only be performed with simultaneous breast reconstruction to fill out the shape left beneath the remaining skin envelope. With nipple-sparing mastectomy, it's important to know that even though the skin of the nipple is preserved and the nipple looks unchanged, sensation is not preserved, as most of the nerve endings leading up to the nipple are cut.

After any type of mastectomy surgery, with or without reconstruction, one or more drains are usually left in place under the skin. A drain is a rubber tube with small perforations that is threaded through a small hole in the skin. We insert the drain so that the fluid that the body makes as part of the healing process does not pool in the empty space that is left behind after the breast has been removed. The tube connects to a small bulb that is squeezed, producing a suction effect that pulls the fluid out of the body into the bulb reservoir. During the postoperative period, the bulb fills up with fluid a few times a day and needs to be emptied, either in the hospital or while you are at home. These drains are usually left in place for a week or more after surgery, and are easily removed in the doctor's office once the amount of fluid coming out tapers off and the drain is no longer needed.

All procedures will have pluses and minuses, and following are those associated with both of these operations. These are the things you need to focus on and discuss when making your decision.

Lumpectomy: advantages and disadvantages

Lumpectomy is one choice for surgery for both DCIS and invasive cancer, and most women are eligible for lumpectomy coupled with subsequent radiation treatment. In fact, in the modern era most cancers detected are small, singular, and well suited for lumpectomy.

Advantage #1: The main advantage to lumpectomy is cosmetic. Even the most masterfully reconstructed breast cannot approximate the result achieved by keeping the existing breast with a small incision. With lumpectomy, the breast usually will look close to the same in size and shape as it did before the surgery, but there will be a scar on the skin somewhere on the breast. Most women heal quite well, and the scar fades and becomes unnoticeable. In addition, an experienced breast surgeon will know how to strategically place the incision so that the scar is less noticeable, without compromising the removal of the cancer.

Advantage #2: Another chief advantage of choosing lumpectomy is that it's a much smaller, shorter operation, and it's usually performed as an outpatient procedure under light anesthesia. The limited nature of the surgery means that there's less healing time and recovery is rapid (similar to the time it takes to heal from stitches for a wound). You'll feel tender for a bit and the stitches in your breast will mean your movements need to be somewhat restricted, but many women return to their jobs, home activities, and regular lives within days of surgery. I have some highly motivated patients who actually show up at work the day after surgery, although I don't usually recommend this. I don't care what you do in life—if you are having surgery, you deserve a few days off! You will also need to adjust your exercise regimen for a couple of weeks as you wait to fully heal.

Disadvantage #1: One of the main disadvantages of lumpectomy is that you *may* have to come back for further surgery. When the surgeon removes the cancer during lumpectomy, he or she is also removing some of the tissue surrounding the cancer in order to ensure clear margins (see chapter 8 for more information on margins). Most cancers aren't shaped like a ball; instead they grow in a star shape with irregular tentacles that extend into the surrounding tissue. When the surgeon takes out the cancer, he or she also removes some tissue around the cancer in order to include those tentacles or extensions as well. Unfortunately, during surgery the surgeon cannot see or feel the exact extent of the cancer and thus has to estimate how much tissue needs to be removed. It's only *after* surgery, when the tissue is sent to the lab for analysis, that we can tell if the margins are clear or not. This happens approximately one week after surgery when the results are reported. If the edges around the cancer come back clear (negative margins), we are confident that the mainstay of the cancer has been removed and no further surgery is needed. When the tissue comes back showing cancer cells at the edge or margin (positive margins), the concern is that there is cancer still left in the breast as well; you may have to return for additional surgery (another lumpectomy or mastectomy) so that more tissue can be removed. This eventuality is quite common— approximately 10 to 20 percent of women who undergo lumpectomy will need additional surgery. Very occasionally, after a lumpectomy is done, the results from the lab show that the cancer is much more extensive than was originally thought. In these cases, mastectomy may be recommended to fully remove the cancer.

Disadvantage #2: In almost all cases, lumpectomy is followed by radiation treatments given over a period of about a month. The idea is that the radiation "mops up" any microscopic cancer cells left behind in the remaining breast after surgery. Your treatment will consist of short bursts of radiation given five days a week for either three or six weeks—which means daily trips to the doctor's office or clinic, and the inconvenience involved in that. Although there are newer types of radiation that may be as effective and that can be given over a shorter course, five days or so, long-term study results do not yet clearly demonstrate that the shorter treatment is as effective in reducing the risk of cancer coming back in the breast. The appropriateness of using these shorter courses of radiation varies from patient to patient. For many women who live in rural areas and would need to travel a great distance for radiation treatment each day, a short course might be the only feasible option. (For information on radiation, go to chapter 10.)

Disadvantage #3: Lumpectomy with radiation is associated with a slightly higher risk of cancer coming back in the breast. The risk of recurrence in the treated breast is quite low—usually less than 5 percent in most cases—but that's still a bit higher than the risk of recurrence associated with mastectomy (1 to 2 percent). It's very important to know that while the risk of recurrence in the breast may be slightly higher with lumpectomy, there is *absolutely no difference* between lumpectomy and mastectomy when it comes to survival rates.

All women who undergo lumpectomy will require future mammograms and often other imaging tests in order to check for recurrence in the breast that was conserved and to check the other breast as well. For some women, this is a cause for anxiety and therefore a disadvantage.

Mastectomy: advantages and disadvantages

Mastectomy is the second option for breast cancer surgery, and as with lumpectomy, is performed for women with both DCIS and invasive cancer.

The advantages and disadvantages of mastectomy are basically opposite those described for lumpectomy:

Advantage #1: Mastectomy is associated with a slightly lower risk of cancer coming back in the breast and chest wall area when compared to a lumpectomy. This makes sense: the less tissue remaining, the less likelihood of developing a new problem in the remaining tissue in the future. A common misconception, however, is that mastectomy *totally* eliminates the chance of a recurrence. In fact, the cancer *can* still come back after a mastectomy, whether it's in the scar tissue or within the minuscule amount of remaining breast tissue. The risks are very low—1 to 2 percent—but it does happen. (Survival rates with the two surgeries, lumpectomy and mastectomy, are identical, as mentioned above.)

Advantage #2: Whereas radiation is almost always given after lumpectomy, mastectomy patients do not generally receive radiation. It makes sense if you think about it: the purpose of radiation is to "mop up" microscopic cells that may be left behind in the breast; however, if the whole breast is removed and there is virtually no tissue left, then there's nothing left to radiate. So if patients are unwilling or unable to receive radiation, mastectomy is usually recommended. (Go to chapter 10 for more on radiation and when it may not be possible.)

Advantage #3: Whereas lumpectomy is associated with a possible need for additional surgery, another advantage of mastectomy is that *all* the breast tissue is removed in one operation, thereby virtually eliminating the need for additional surgery. So if you don't want to risk undergoing multiple successive procedures, mastectomy may be the best option.

Advantage #4: One of the most frequently cited reasons for choosing mastectomy is that it eliminates the need for future imaging such as mammograms, sonograms, and MRIs. When mastectomy is performed, there is no role for future imaging of the breast, because virtually no breast tissue remains. Obviously, this isn't the case for patients who have undergone a lumpectomy and who still have to undergo regular screening. Many women express significant anxiety when it comes to facing future tests, the results, and the possible need for future biopsies. For these women, the emotional toll of subsequent mammograms, sonograms, or MRIs is so high that they opt for mastectomy.

Disadvantage #1: Lumpectomy is a smaller operation usually associated with a quick recovery. Mastectomy, on the other hand, is a larger operation with a longer recovery period, and usually involves a stay in the hospital; the length of the stay depends on where you have your surgery and what type of reconstruction is involved. While many women are up and around the day of mastectomy surgery, they still are quite limited in their overall activity, and usually require more pain medication postoperatively than do lumpectomy patients. In addition, while the most extensive part of reconstruction is usually performed at the same time as the mastectomy, the majority of reconstruction procedures are performed in phases and are not complete after just one operation, so there is usually more than one procedure to recover from. (For more on reconstruction, see chapter 7.)

Disadvantage #2: Mastectomy is associated with more disfigurement than lumpectomy is, for obvious reasons, especially if no reconstruction is performed. Even with reconstruction, many women will lose the nipple and the sensation in that area, so mastectomy is associated with a significant amount of numbness along the chest wall. Newer options for mastectomy that can save the nipple are increasingly being offered, but they are not appropriate for everyone, and even when the nipple is saved, the sensation in the nipple is lost.

Advantage/disadvantage: Many women who do choose mastectomy decide to have breast reconstruction done at the same time. On the downside, this can further extend the recovery time for many patients, and let's face it—a reconstructed breast will not perfectly match the look, feel, or sensation of your original breast. On the upside, significant improvements in reconstructive options and techniques mean that your new breast (or breasts) will likely look more natural than reconstructed breasts did in decades past. And for some women who aren't happy with the size or shape of their natural breasts, breast reconstruction after cancer surgery not only helps cushion the blow of losing your breast but also can be a silver lining, helping you get the breasts you *really* wanted through reconstruction.

NEED TO KNOW

It's critically important to know that having a mastectomy and reconstruction is not at all like having breast implants and should never be thought of that way: adding an implant to one's own breast is totally different from removing one's own breast tissue and putting an implant in to fill the empty space. But for many women, having reconstruction definitely makes the option of mastectomy more appealing.

In essence, the main disadvantages of mastectomy are that you have to undergo a bigger operation that has more significant ramifications for overall appearance and cosmetic outcome, loss of sensation and function, and a longer path to full recovery.

MYTH: "If you have a mastectomy, you will live longer."
If you *are* given the choice by your surgeon between lumpectomy and mastectomy, here is the most critical piece of information you will need to help inform your decision: *there is absolutely no difference whatsoever in survival when comparing the two surgeries.* None whatsoever. And

yet the vast majority of women arriving at my office bring with them the misconception that the more extensive surgery, mastectomy, is a more aggressive way of fighting the disease, and therefore translates to a higher chance of survival.

Nothing could be further from the truth. Survival from breast cancer has *nothing* to do with how much tissue you remove from the diseased breast. Survival from breast cancer has everything to do with how much *cancer* you remove (ideally, all of it). If the cancer is small and can be taken out with a lumpectomy, then removing additional healthy breast tissue does not give you a survival advantage in any way. When cancer spreads to other parts of the body, this spread (metastasis) occurs *prior* to the surgery, before anyone knows that a cancer is present, when microscopic cancer cells break off from the tumor in the breast and circulate in the bloodstream. When this happens, chemotherapy can often eradicate this microscopic disease, but it is not always successful in doing so. How much breast tissue you decide to remove really has no effect on microscopic cells that may have already broken off and started to spread. That's why more extensive surgery on the breast has no greater effect on survival.

Yet many women persist in believing that mastectomy will improve their odds. You don't have to look far to find the source of this misinformation: there's a chorus of voices on the Internet repeating this inaccurate assertion over and over. Most are well-meaning or are the voices of women who chose mastectomy because they, like so many, couldn't abide the idea of leaving breast tissue behind that could potentially harbor or develop cancer again in the future. This leap of logic is totally understandable—many people can't stand the thought of leaving in place tissue and thus cells that have already proven they can develop into cancer. Even for normal surrounding breast tissue and the other breast, there is "guilt by association," leading to the assumption that removing it all will provide you with some peace of mind. But it's worth repeating one more time: there is absolutely no difference whatsoever in survival when comparing the two surgeries. None whatsoever.

Personal versus medical factors in your decision making

If you are like most women with newly diagnosed breast cancer, you will have two equal options: mastectomy and lumpectomy with radiation. The advantages and disadvantages discussed above are part of *personal* decision making and preferences that may influence your choices. But there are some *medical* factors that may influence decision making and would therefore be factored into the recommendation made by the surgeon advising you.

When lumpectomy isn't possible

There are four main reasons why lumpectomy may not be a viable option:

1. When there is a large cancer (typically greater than four to five centimeters, or approximately two inches) it may be difficult to remove the whole tumor, along with its margins, with a lumpectomy without leaving the patient with a result that's disfiguring. For women with larger breasts, larger tumors may still be amenable to lumpectomy, depending on the ratio of tumor size to breast size. Your surgeon's job is to guide you in decision making by giving you information about what is technically feasible, given your individual breast and tumor sizes, and by giving you a realistic idea as to what the cosmetic result might look like if you would prefer lumpectomy. And there is one caveat: if you do want a lumpectomy and your tumor is on the larger side, you may want to ask your doctor whether having chemotherapy first might shrink the tumor and improve your chances of having a successful lumpectomy. This strategy is not appropriate in all cases, but it may be worth discussing with your surgeon. (For more on this, see chapter 9 on neoadjuvant chemotherapy.)

2. When there are two or more separate tumors in the breast, this usually warrants a mastectomy. How far apart do these tumors have to be to be considered separate? Again, it depends on breast size, location of the tumors in the breast, and whether or not the

surgeon feels that he or she can remove the two cancers, get a clear margin around them, and leave you with a satisfying cosmetic result. Your surgeon should help you determine if this is a viable option. Occasionally a double lumpectomy can be performed, but it is currently not the standard of care.

3. Cancers that involve the nipple are often, but not always, better served with mastectomy and reconstruction of the breast and nipple. Because the nipple is such a cosmetically focal part of the breast, it is often difficult to remove the nipple and leave a woman with a pleasing cosmetic result. In addition, many women with cancers that involve the nipple may also have a significant amount of cancer behind the nipple and thus would require the removal of the whole central part of the breast. The cosmetic result after such a lumpectomy is usually not very satisfactory, and mastectomy with reconstruction may be a better choice in this scenario.

4. When patients have had prior radiation to either the breast or chest wall, lumpectomy is not the recommended choice. The skin and soft tissue in any area cannot tolerate more than one round of radiation treatment, and as radiation is almost always given in tandem with lumpectomy, this type of surgery is no longer an option for patients who have undergone radiation in the past. So if a woman has had a prior lumpectomy and radiation and the cancer recurs, mastectomy is the treatment of choice. Many women use this fact to rationalize turning down radiation to treat their cancer the first time around, so that if it recurs, they are still candidates for lumpectomy *with* radiation if, heaven forbid, there is a second time. The problem with this line of thinking is that *without* radiation the first time, the risk of the cancer coming back *is* much higher, so the situation becomes a self-fulfilling prophecy. In most cases the recommendation is to have radiation coupled with the lumpectomy at first diagnosis, understanding that if the cancer comes back despite this full treatment, mastectomy is the best option.

5. Morbidly obese women may not be able to have a lumpectomy, as many radiation tables have a weight limit of approximately

300 to 350 pounds. If you can't have the radiation to follow, in most cases you can't have a lumpectomy.

6. Lumpectomy is usually *not* advised when patients are genetically predisposed to cancer, because with lumpectomy alone, there is a higher likelihood of cancer coming back or a new one developing in the same or the opposite breast. (See chapter 15 for more on genetic predisposition to breast cancer.) In such cases of genetic predisposition, your surgeon may recommend a mastectomy or even double mastectomy, especially for a woman who is young (in her twenties, thirties, or forties) at the time of her first diagnosis.

When lumpectomy is actively recommended

For patients who are elderly or infirm, lumpectomy may be the better option, as the surgery is shorter and less extensive and can often be done under a lighter anesthesia. In general, the lumpectomy is associated with lower operative risk and quicker recovery from surgery for people who are older or not in the best of health.

When radiation may not be necessary after lumpectomy

A minority of women may not require radiation after lumpectomy (for more on radiation see chapter 10). Recent studies show that women who are over the age of seventy with smaller cancers that respond well to hormone treatment may not need radiation in addition to surgery and hormonal treatment, and have a very low risk of cancer coming back in the breast with lumpectomy alone. The safety of omitting radiation needs to be determined on a case-by-case basis by breast specialists.

MAKING THE DECISION: WHEN YOU HAVE EQUAL OPTIONS

Once it has been established that you are a candidate for either lumpectomy or mastectomy, then the choice between the two is no longer a medical decision but a personal one. If your doctor gives you a choice and asks you which surgery you would prefer, it's not a trick question. There is no single right answer for everyone. Your doctor is asking you to make the decision that is *right for you*. Only you can know which option suits you the best.

The very personalized nature of this decision became clear to me early on in my practice as a surgeon, when on the same day I met with two women with seemingly identical backgrounds and cases who had very different reactions when it came to making choices about their respective surgical options. Carolyn, in her mid-thirties, was the mother of two young children, an investment banker, and a candidate for both lumpectomy and mastectomy. After examining her and reviewing her mammogram, I discussed the options. Midway through our conversation, Carolyn looked at me with clear conviction and said, "If a lumpectomy and mastectomy are associated with equal survival, why would anyone want a mastectomy? I have two young daughters, and as long as you're telling me survival is the same, I want to recover as quickly as I can and get back to my crazy, busy life as soon as possible. What's more, I want to look as normal as possible, and for my girls to see that I have a normal anatomy as they grow up." This made perfect sense to me, and she went on to have a successful lumpectomy.

Later that very same day, another young woman, Alison, came into my office. She was also newly diagnosed with breast cancer, and her profile was remarkably similar to that of Carolyn: she was in her thirties, had two young children, worked in the financial sector, and also had a small cancer amenable to lumpectomy. As I started discussing the options, Alison stopped me. "Wait a minute," she said. "I know that you said that lumpectomy and mastectomy are associated with the same survival rates, and I know the likelihood of developing a new cancer on the other side is low, but I want the *lowest* risk—I want a double mastectomy. I also don't want to live in fear of my annual mammogram, and I never really liked the way my breasts looked anyway."

This made perfect sense to me too. These two women, similar in many ways, chose two diametrically opposed surgical approaches. Each one made the appropriate decision for herself, her life, and her future.

So after your surgeon offers you appropriate options from a medical standpoint, it is up to you to decide what the best choice is from a *personal* standpoint. There's no question that this can be one of the most complicated and significant decisions a woman will have to make in her lifetime. For most of the patients I see at my office, it's a question of weighing all the contributing factors as carefully as possible. A fifty-eight-year-old woman who is diagnosed while going through a divorce and who is thinking about returning to the world of dating at some point may make a different decision than a forty-year-old woman who is in a stable relationship and in the midst of bringing up young children. And it's hard to predict what decision any individual will make until she is actually in the situation and has to make the choice for herself. I always tell my patients: "I may be the expert on breast cancer, but you're the expert on *you.*"

MYTH: "If you have a mastectomy, you won't need any treatment after surgery."

When making the decision of lumpectomy versus mastectomy, some women lean toward a mastectomy under the mistaken belief that it means they can avoid additional treatment after surgery. While it's true that radiation is almost always given with lumpectomy and not commonly given with a mastectomy unless there is more advanced disease, it's important to keep in mind that a mastectomy does not eliminate the possibility that you might need additional chemotherapy after surgery. A woman who needs chemotherapy after a lumpectomy also needs it after a mastectomy: the same kind and the same amount. So if you are making a decision about surgery, don't choose a mastectomy with the idea that you will avoid additional treatment.

MYTH: "If cancer has spread to the lymph nodes, then mastectomy is a better choice than lumpectomy."

Huge misconception and positively not true. Having positive lymph nodes may mean that more lymph nodes need to be removed, but it does *not* mean that more tissue needs to be taken from the breast. As long as lumpectomy with clear margins can be achieved in the same way that we would desire for a woman with negative nodes, lumpectomy is perfectly acceptable for women with positive nodes.

Tuning out the background noise

If you are given a choice of surgery, this is as important a time as any to tune out the background noise. This is a decision best made in collaboration with your doctor and those people closest to you. It's not a decision that can be easily made by polling your wider community or in consultation with strangers you've met in Internet chat rooms. Sometimes it's comforting and helpful when strangers call and email to share their experiences and give advice. Women who previously had breast cancer themselves, a sorority of survivors, offer to share their stories, and some are even willing to show you the results from their surgery. Remember that the decisions they made and their stories may or may not be applicable to your decisions and your story. And if anyone who has *not* had breast cancer has the audacity to say to you, "If I were in your position, I would [fill in the blank]," you have every right to ignore that person. No one, including myself, knows what kind of decision she would make when faced with such a choice, and it is presumptuous to assume otherwise.

Lumpectomy versus mastectomy: issues that *don't* factor in

Every patient who walks into my office comes with a list of questions. Many of these questions are vital and need to be addressed. You need to understand what is going on, and you need to know how to ask whether your doctors have the necessary experience to perform your surgery successfully. Then there are those questions that people outside the medical field may tell you to ask but which are not at all relevant when it comes to deciding between a mastectomy and a lumpectomy. I hear these questions every day, and I think it's important to address the three most common ones and explain why asking them will *not* help your decision making.

1. **What stage am I?** Patients frequently come into the surgeon's office right after they have received their diagnosis. Their first question is usually "Doctor, what stage am I?" If they have had a needle biopsy, the answer from the surgeon should be "I don't know yet." The surgeon can make an educated guess at this point, but the true stage is not definitively determined until after surgery, when the pathology report is available. The staging of the cancer depends mainly on two factors: lymph node status and tumor size. Although we can estimate tumor size early in the process (for example, a biopsy that shows DCIS most likely means stage 0 breast cancer), other factors that may contribute information about stage (such as lymph node status) can often be determined only after obtaining results from surgery. Because the surgeon cannot really provide definitive information about staging beforehand, the stage of your cancer will usually not be a factor in your decision. And more important, for most women the stage of their cancer will *not* change the recommendation for lumpectomy or mastectomy. If a woman has a small tumor but spread to the lymph nodes is found, this brings her to stage 2 instead of stage 1. But in and of itself, having lymph node spread does not mean that more tissue needs to be taken from the breast or that a mastectomy would be a better choice.

2. **How long has my cancer been there and how fast is it growing?** In general, cancers grow slowly, over the course of months or years, not days or weeks. Usually they are treated soon after they are detected. The only way of truly knowing how quickly a cancer is growing is by *not* treating it, then checking back a few months later to see what has happened. Did it grow a little bit in size? Did it double? Most people, thankfully, do not choose this course. So for most women there is no way of knowing how rapidly a particular cancer is growing. Many women feel as though their cancers just "popped up" out of nowhere and so are understandably concerned that the cancer is growing very quickly. One day they were in the shower washing and felt a mass, whereas the previous day they didn't. There is no question that there is always a single day, a single moment when the cancer is first no-

ticed, but even if it seems as if it appeared suddenly, it has certainly been there for some time. Either it's a slow-growing cancer and has been there for a long time or it's a fast-growing cancer that has been there for a shorter time. There is no way for anyone to know whether your cancer is slow- or fast-growing unless we simply wait and see. Therefore your surgical decisions can't depend on this factor.

3. **What would you do if you were me?** Whenever a patient asks me this question, I always tell them that what *I* would do in the situation actually isn't relevant to their case. Here's why. Ultimately, only you can decide from your own perspective, and when the options are medically equal, your surgeon's perspective shouldn't really factor in to your decision. As an experienced breast specialist, I can only offer my patients good options; there is no wrong choice, only the right choice for *you*. Your surgeon can never truly walk in your shoes or experience your life from your perspective. As a surgeon, I might be the type of person who wants to get back to work as soon as possible and thus would choose the smallest possible operation with the shortest recovery time. You might be someone who would rather have a longer recovery time than have to go back to a regular screening regimen. Everyone's story is different, and the choice is ultimately yours and yours alone. The only thing that might be helpful to know is that in the United States, most women who are eligible to have a lumpectomy choose to do so.

MYTH: "The majority of women get mastectomies, so that must be the better option."

This is a very common misconception. In fact, it's untrue on both counts. First, the majority of women with breast cancer get lumpectomies, *not* mastectomies. Second, there is no difference in survival rates between lumpectomy with radiation and mastectomy.

Why is this myth so pervasive, especially online? My guess is that women who undergo lumpectomy are something of a silent majority. They tend to have their surgery and move on. These women generally don't have to stay in the hospital and their recovery time is minimal, so they often get back to their normal activities earlier, with less interruption to their usual routine. They may not need to tell a large circle of people about their diagnosis and/or surgery—and as a result, you're less likely to hear their survivor stories.

By contrast, women receiving mastectomies are much more likely to share with a wider group because their surgery is more extensive, recovery time is longer, and they may have a greater need to inform friends and work colleagues about what's happening to them. It follows that these women may be more vocal about their breast cancer and disproportionately represented among those sharing their survivor stories in your community, on the Internet, in chat rooms, or on advocacy sites. A vicious cycle has been created where the *perception* is that mastectomy is the better and more widely chosen option, leading some women to choose more extensive surgery when they could have had a more minimal one without altering their survival chances in any way.

WHAT ABOUT THE OTHER BREAST?

In recent years, more and more women who require or choose a mastectomy in one breast are choosing to have bilateral or double mastectomies (opting to remove the other, healthy breast as well as the breast with cancer). Why has there been such an upsurge in numbers of bilateral mastectomies? It seems to be related to a few different factors:

1. Modern plastic surgery has developed techniques that offer women much better cosmetic results, and so the option of removing both breasts has become much less terrifying than it was in decades past. (For more on reconstruction, see chapter 7.) For some women there will be an aesthetic benefit when both breasts are removed, as the outcome is likely to be more symmetrical, especially for women with pendulous, hanging breasts; these women might otherwise require surgery to lift the normal breast in order to achieve a matched result.

2. The increased use of MRI screening has led to increased numbers of abnormalities being identified in the second breast. Occasionally the abnormalities that are seen are truly cancer that

would not otherwise have been detected, but far more frequently the findings are actually false positives, something that has been seen but is *not* cancer (for more on screening and false positives, see chapter 1). The problem with false positive results is that the only way to differentiate a true finding from a false positive is to perform a biopsy. Additional biopsies often delay surgery, lead to increased anxiety, and result in a seemingly endless stream of additional tests. Rather than go through with this level of intervention, many women elect to remove the other breast regardless of whether the finding proves to be cancer. This course of action also serves the secondary purpose of eliminating the need for any future imaging.

3. Thanks to genetic testing, we now know that there is a small group of women with breast cancer who *are* at significantly higher risk of getting a new cancer in the other breast, and for this specific group of women, removing the other breast is often advisable. (See chapter 15, on genetic predisposition.)

MYTH: "Removing the normal breast along with the breast with cancer improves your chances of survival."

This is simply not true. In the worst-case scenario that the breast cancer does come back, it typically spreads to other parts of the body. Although women with breast cancer *can* develop a new cancer in the other breast, breast cancer in one breast *does not* spread to the other breast. You may be surprised to learn that for most women with breast cancer the likelihood of developing a new cancer in the other breast is extremely low: usually under 5 percent over the ensuing ten years. So leaving the healthy breast in place after cancer has been found does not present a particularly high risk for development of a new cancer in the other breast down the line.

Also remember that with every intervention there is risk. While breast surgery is generally well tolerated and the serious risks are low, there are potential complications with all surgical procedures (bleeding, infection, and the risk of anesthesia, to name a few). The longer and more extensive an operation is, the greater the risk. So removal of the other breast is not a free ride. *Any* complication in surgery, especially infection, could delay future treatment that is needed for the known cancer. Sometimes if the cancer is known to be particularly aggressive—perhaps there is a large mass or multiple lymph nodes involved—a surgeon may recommend *against* doing a mastectomy on the unaffected breast. This way your doctors can remain focused on the significant problem at hand—the known high-risk cancer—without the potential complication of additional surgery on the other side, especially as there is no survival benefit to the removal of the second breast.

Removing the other breast: the role of anxiety

Often women who are considering removing the other (healthy) breast are considering doing so not simply to reduce risk but also to reduce anxiety. It's very common for women to feel fearful about developing a new cancer on the other side, even if the risk is small. This can lead to anxiety around the need for future mammograms, MRIs, or biopsies. Women who feel this way often feel compelled to do anything and everything that can possibly be done to reduce the risk of ever having to deal with breast cancer again.

Anxiety, however, is a complicated emotion. For some women, it's specific and brought on by a certain situation or circumstance. For others, it is a general state of existence—they always veer to a more anxious state of mind. I have many patients who choose to remove the other breast because they don't want to face the emotional stress of future tests. Then, six months after surgery, they come into my office concerned about their future risk of ovarian cancer, asking for a referral to see a specialist to remove their ovaries. And by the way, shouldn't they also be getting a colonoscopy earlier than recommended too? Some women just have very anxious personalities. The problem is, you can't just keep removing body parts in order to allay anxiety.

If you do have an anxious mind-set, it is important to be honest with yourself. Are you making decisions designed to eliminate anxiety, when the reality is that even if you remove both breasts you will find some new focus of concern and still end up feeling fearful? My advice is to take the time you need to fully consider what you are trying to accomplish by removing the other breast, and to be clear about whether removing the other breast will truly achieve that purpose.

A FEW SPECIAL SITUATIONS: WHEN DIFFERENT TREATMENT OPTIONS ARE CONSIDERED

Bilateral breast cancer

A very small number of women—approximately 1 percent of patients with newly diagnosed breast cancer—will have breast cancer in both breasts. It's important to know that this is *not* because the cancer has spread from one side to the other. It's because these are two separate cancers that happen to have developed in tandem. Usually the diagnosis of bilateral breast cancer happens after diagnosis on one side leads to additional imaging, such as an MRI, which then identifies something on the other side that when biopsied proves to be cancer.

Bilateral breast cancer involves some special considerations to factor into your decision making process for surgery.

1. If your surgeon confirms that lumpectomy can be done on both sides, this is certainly reasonable to do. But there is often a higher risk of needing more surgery as a result of needing to get clear margins on *both* sides, not just one. While radiation cannot be given to the *same* breast twice, radiation *can* be given to each breast individually following bilateral lumpectomy.
2. Women who need a mastectomy on one side but can have a lumpectomy on the other may choose to do this, but then they will still need radiation for the lumpectomy side, as well as future imaging. Many women with bilateral breast cancer who *need* a mastectomy on one side often end up choosing to have a mastectomy for both.
3. Overall staging is based on which side is the most advanced. For example, a woman with DCIS in one breast (stage 0) and a small invasive cancer with normal nodes on the other (stage 1) would

be considered stage 1. Decision making for subsequent treatment would be based on the cancer that is most advanced.

4. If you are diagnosed with bilateral breast cancer, especially at a young age, you may want to consider genetic testing prior to deciding what kind of surgery to have. Genetic predisposition could indicate an increased risk of the cancer coming back again, on either side, which could then lead you to choose more extensive surgery, even when lumpectomy on both sides may be feasible. (See chapter 15 for further information on the BRCA genes, genetic testing, and the implications for surgical decision making.)

Treatment of occult breast cancer

For women with occult breast cancer (see chapter 5), where the breast tumor is not seen on mammogram or felt on examination and the first sign of it was a cancerous lymph node in the armpit, treatment options depend specifically on whether further investigation is able to find the actual cancer in the breast. The test of choice for identifying an occult cancer in the breast is an MRI, which does identify the culprit in approximately 70 percent of cases. If the cancer in the breast is found, then treatment can proceed as usual, with options of lumpectomy and mastectomy based on the usual criteria. When the source of cancer in the breast (also called the primary tumor) cannot be identified within the breast even after MRI, clearly a lumpectomy cannot be done on an area that cannot be found. Options for treatment in this setting include mastectomy or just radiation treatment to the breast without its removal. In both cases lymph nodes are removed with axillary dissection as a result of known spread, which was how the cancer was identified in the first place.

Inflammatory breast cancer: a rare, aggressive cancer that needs us to be aggressive back

Inflammatory breast cancer is a rare, aggressive type of breast cancer that not only involves the whole breast and lymph nodes but usually involves a significant portion of the overlying breast skin as well. Treatment of inflammatory breast cancer requires chemotherapy first in order to shrink the cancer and reduce the skin involvement. With a good response to chemotherapy, mastectomy is subsequently performed to remove whatever disease is left. Lumpectomy is never an option for a woman with inflammatory breast cancer, even if it appears as though the cancer shrank considerably. For this rare but particularly aggressive form of breast cancer, radiation is also needed, even after mastectomy. Historically the prognosis for inflammatory breast cancer was quite grim. But with the combination of aggressive modern-day treatment options—chemotherapy, surgery, and radiation—even for this rare type of cancer there is room for optimism and the possibility of cure.

Paget's disease

Paget's disease is another rare form of breast cancer. It starts in the nipple and is essentially treated the same way as other subtypes of breast cancer. However, removal of the nipple is part of the treatment for Paget's disease. The decision to perform a lumpectomy or mastectomy is usually based on how much cancer, in addition to the nipple, is present in the rest of the breast. As with any standard lumpectomy, radiation is usually required for Paget's disease when lumpectomy is selected.

Additional testing before surgery

After a cancer diagnosis but before any surgery is done, there's always the question of whether or not additional tests are needed. Some tests, like MRI, look at the breasts to determine if any other areas of cancer in either breast can be identified now that one has been diagnosed. Other tests, like CT, bone, and PET scans, look at the entire body to determine if the cancer has spread.

There are various considerations that need to be taken into account when considering additional tests. Again, one approach does not fit all cases. The key is individualization and deciding which tests are appropriate for each *specific* situation. As you work with your surgeon to determine what, if any, additional tests you need before your surgery, there are considerations to keep in mind. Some physicians believe that every woman with breast cancer should have scans of her body to determine if the cancer has spread. But for the majority of patients with a new diagnosis of breast cancer, there really is no reason to do this, and national guidelines recommend against it.

In general, we only want to order further scans when there are specific symptoms leading a physician to suspect metastasis or spread of the disease. Some of these symptoms include—but are not limited to—new bone pain, neurologic symptoms such as blurry vision or loss of consciousness, or new abdominal pain or jaundice. There are other cases where checking the body for spread before proceeding with surgery should be done, since finding that the cancer has spread could strongly impact plans for treatment. For example, if your breast cancer has been shown to have substantial spread to the lymph nodes under the arm, your doctor may want to check with scans to make sure the cancer has not taken the next step beyond that, to other parts of the body.

Outside of these circumstances, there are clear-cut research and data that show that for women with breast cancer who have smaller tumors and no symptoms or signs of spread, scans of the body done before surgery will demonstrate cancer spread *less than 1 percent of the time.* You may say, "So what? If I am in the 1 percent, I want to know. And besides, what's the harm? More information must always be better, right?" Wrong. In general, more is not always better, and there are serious potential consequences that can result from every test we do. The more you look, the more you find. And in most situations with an early breast cancer diagnosis, what you find is more likely to be normal—a false positive—than to be something that is actually significant. The only way to know for sure if a particular finding is normal or not is to do a biopsy of the newly found spot. And doing a biopsy in some obscure site in the body can take time, delay the treatment of the breast cancer, and lead to additional stress and anxiety for you. Biopsies can also be associated with their own set of complications. A biopsy of the lung, for instance, can lead to collapse of that lung. A biopsy of the liver could result in life-threatening bleeding. So the decision to do additional scans can come with a price.

Sometimes additional tests are ordered by a woman's general doctor or gynecologist, who is directing care before she has even seen the surgeon. But recent data has also shown that even some oncologists "over order" scans of the body looking for spread when it's not really indicated. A surgeon or oncologist who specializes in breast cancer is usually familiar with the rationale behind appropriate test selection. When you do meet with your surgeon, you should have a thoughtful discussion about what, if any, additional tests need to be done prior to proceeding with surgery or treatment. But remember, in most cases additional scans are not necessary, more does not mean better, and a doctor who orders lots of tests is not necessarily more thorough than one who doesn't.

THE TAKEAWAY

- Lumpectomy with radiation and mastectomy—these two options are associated with equivalent survival rates. Keep this at the forefront of your mind when making your decision.
- Think carefully about the decision to remove the other breast. It won't prevent the cancer from coming back, and it is not associated with improved survival. It may give you a more symmetrical aesthetic result, however, and will eliminate the need for future mammograms and other imaging tests.
- There is no one-size-fits-all approach when it comes to additional testing.

CHAPTER 7

Reconstruction

better options than ever before

M ost women who have mastectomies, particularly in younger age groups, choose to undergo reconstruction. While it is not required by any means, reconstruction has been shown to greatly improve quality of life, self-image, and overall well-being for many women who have mastectomies. Reconstruction is rarely needed or performed after a lumpectomy.

Reconstructive surgery is usually performed in stages, with the first stage happening at the same time as the mastectomy surgery, when the breast is removed. This means that when a woman wakes up from surgery, she has some semblance of a reconstructed breast and does not have to look at a flat chest wall. Usually the rest of the stages of reconstruction happen weeks to months later, depending on whether additional treatment is needed; for example, if chemotherapy is given after surgery, the second stage of reconstruction would wait until after chemotherapy has been completed. If you decide not to have reconstruction at the time of your mastectomy and then change your mind after surgery is done, reconstruction usually can be performed at a later time, but there are advantages to doing it at the same time as the mastectomy. For one, if you do reconstruction later, you would need an extra operation that could have been combined with your breast surgery. For another, in some cases other treatments you receive—specifically radiation, which is given after mastectomy in cases of advanced breast cancer—can make reconstruction more challenging afterward and limit your options (for more on this, see chapter 10 and below). So if you are considering reconstruction, having it at the same time as your breast surgery is usually the best way to go.

There are situations where your breast surgeon may actually recommend *against* reconstruction. One is in rare cases of very advanced breast cancer, such as inflammatory breast cancer. While complications related to reconstruction are not common, they do happen, and in cases of more advanced disease, your surgeon may be concerned that *any* complication could delay cancer treatment that is critically needed right away. Another involves women who have other major health issues; the surgeon may feel that the additional hours of surgery needed to perform reconstruction would be too risky. In these cases, focusing only on the goal of curing the cancer may be the best plan.

Reconstruction is usually performed by a plastic surgeon working closely with the breast surgeon to achieve the best combined result for both cancer cure and aesthetics. When you opt for reconstruction at the same time as your mastectomy your plastic surgeon and breast surgeon have to work together, and thus both have to be affiliated with the institution or facility where your surgery will be performed. So usually your breast surgeon will refer you to a plastic surgeon that he or she works with regularly. Most breast surgeons do work with more than one plastic surgeon, so you can ask your breast surgeon about the different options for referral, and you may even want to consult with more than one. (Also see chapter 4 on putting together your team.) You will meet with the plastic surgeon for a consultation prior to surgery, and during that visit you will be examined and options for reconstruction for you will be discussed. Many plastic surgeons will show you pictures of their previous work as examples of results they have achieved, but remember, each patient is different, and her results will depend on many contributing factors, including body type, overall health, and other factors related to her particular case. Once you have met your plastic surgeon and decided on your surgery team, the two doctors' offices will usually work together to coordinate a surgery date for you.

In this day and age, reconstructive options are more varied and promising and associated with better cosmetic outcomes than ever before. For each individual woman there may be different options regarding where to make the incision, choices for shape and size of the reconstructed breast, and for some the option of preserving the nipple. Your breast surgeon and plastic surgeon work together harmoniously to maximize your cosmetic outcome while making sure the cancer outcome is the best it can be.

There are two types of breast reconstruction: implant surgery and autologous tissue surgery, known as tissue reconstruction. Each approach has its own advantages and disadvantages.

Implant surgery

In general, implant surgery is the most common way of reconstructing breasts after a mastectomy. It is faster than tissue reconstruction, usually adding two to four hours to the mastectomy surgery (depending on whether the plastic surgeon is reconstructing one or two breasts). Further, the recovery time is similar to just mastectomy alone. Even on the day of surgery, a woman who has had a bilateral mastectomy with implant reconstruction can be up and around, using the bathroom by herself, and starting to drink and eat.

The downside of implant surgery is that you will usually need additional procedures. At the time of mastectomy surgery the first stage of reconstruction is performed by the plastic surgeon: a temporary device, called a tissue expander, is placed in the chest. This is not the actual permanent implant. Over the next few weeks to months after surgery, the expander is injected with saline to make it larger, thereby stretching the overlying remaining skin until the plastic surgeon feels that there is room for the permanent implant. If you need chemotherapy after surgery, this process of expansion can usually proceed without a problem during that time. A second, smaller operation is then required to exchange the expander for the permanent implant. This can happen soon after the first surgery, perhaps a month or two later, if no additional treatment is given. But if you need chemotherapy, this second stage would wait until after treatment is completed. Finally, there's a third procedure required in order to reconstruct the nipple if that's what you choose to do. Nipple reconstruction involves raising a small mound of skin from the scar, or taking a skin graft from another part of the body (often the inner thigh) to create the shape of the nipple. Then once healing is completed, the darker color of the nipple and surrounding areola is achieved with tattooing. For women who are able to undergo nipple-sparing mastectomy, the nipple reconstruction step is not needed.

In some cases it's possible to have immediate reconstruction—which means going straight to permanent implants at the time of the mastectomy. These cases include women where most of the skin and nipple can be safely saved (so there is enough room for the permanent implant without the expansion process) and where the native breast is similar to what is desired so that no significant alteration in overall breast size and shape needs to be made.

Most women who have reconstruction do undergo implant reconstruction. The options for implant reconstruction have improved dramatically over the years, with different shapes and materials now available for different body types. Implants are made of saline or silicone, and both have long-standing track records for safety. Some newer types of silicone implants give them a softer, more natural feel. But implants aren't for everyone. The fact remains that implants are implants and not one's own tissue, so they may never look and feel as natural as you might have hoped. For women who require radiation after mastectomy (see chapter 10), there is also a higher chance of complications with implants, with extensive capsule formation around the implant leading to potential scarring, distortion, and discomfort. But overall most women are satisfied with their implant-based reconstruction.

Autologous tissue surgery

This second option for reconstruction involves taking tissue (fat and skin) from another part of the body where there is some extra (usually the belly, sometimes the buttock, or even the back) and using that tissue to rebuild the breast shape. One advantage of this surgery is a more natural look and shape. In general, a large amount of the patient's own breast skin can be preserved as an envelope, and the tissue from the other site is used to fill in the empty space and can be sculpted to re-create the original or desired shape.

A second advantage of this surgery is that there are no expanders placed, and therefore no second surgery to replace the expander with the implant, so that's one less procedure you will have to undergo. If your nipple was not preserved in the initial surgery, however, and you want it reconstructed, you will still have to have that follow-up procedure. When tissue is taken from the belly the operation is called DIEP flap surgery. DIEP stands for deep inferior epigastric perforator, which is the name of a blood vessel in the belly wall that serves as the main blood supply for the segment of tissue that is being moved. For women who have enough belly tissue to re-create one or both breasts, a third advantage of the tissue transfer operation is getting a simultaneous tummy tuck along with their breast cancer surgery. When tissue is taken from the back, it involves removal of a small part of the latissimus dorsi muscle, which overlies the shoulder blade, along with some fat and skin, and is thus called a latissimus dorsi flap, or lat flap for short.

The major disadvantage of autologous tissue reconstruction surgery is its length and the associated major recovery required. During surgery, the surgeon meticulously connects the blood vessels of the chest wall with the donor tissue vessels by sewing them together, one at a time, so that the donor tissue will be able to live in the new site. This is a complex and delicate process, frequently performed under a microscope; it can take anywhere from six to twelve hours, and sometimes longer. Recovery time is also affected: tissue has been taken from one site in the body and placed in another area, so you're actually healing from two procedures instead of one. When the belly is the tissue donor site, as is usually the case, the recovery is similar to that of someone recovering from major abdominal surgery. When tissue is taken from the back, there can be some weakness of the shoulder and remaining muscle. Full recovery can take as long as six weeks, and patients are definitely not up and around immediately following surgery, as they are after reconstruction with implants.

Another tough decision: implant or tissue transfer after mastectomy?

The plastic surgeon's job is to evaluate you and your body type and to determine whether reconstruction is for you, and if so, what type of reconstruction is best. There are various reasons a plastic surgeon may advise one type of reconstruction over the other. For example, a woman who has had previous radiation to the breast may not be able to have reconstruction with an implant, since the effects of the radiation may mean that the skin cannot be easily stretched (see chapter 10 on radiation side effects). In that case, you'll likely be advised to go with a tissue transfer procedure. Conversely, a thin woman with no extra abdominal fat or a woman with abdominal scars from previous surgery may not be an appropriate candidate for tissue transfer and will be recommended for an implant.

Perhaps the most difficult part of the plastic surgeon's job is managing patient expectations. When a woman develops breast cancer and opts for mastectomy with reconstruction, she may see it as an opportunity to change the size and conformation of her breasts. For example, a thin woman with very small breasts who always wanted larger breasts can opt for a large implant, and a second implant can also be placed behind the opposite breast to create a match. But if a woman weighs 270 pounds and opts for a belly flap, this will rearrange some of the tissue and put it in more desirable places, but it won't make her 125 pounds. And neither of these women will wake up with a different overall body type.

In other words, be realistic in your expectations. Breast reconstruction has been shown to improve quality of life, self-image, and overall well-being for many women who have a mastectomy, but it is not a total body overhaul. In addition, it's best to be skeptical if the plastic surgeon's promises for physical transformation seem far-fetched or unrealistic.

Oncoplastic surgery

Oncoplastic surgery, which has been buzzed about in the last few years, simply means combining breast cancer surgery (the "onco" part) with

A WORD TO THE WISE

Planning your surgery is best done with a team approach in which a plastic surgeon and breast surgeon who work well together strategize to achieve the best outcome for you. This involves up-front discussion of many different factors about your case (implant versus tissue, preservation versus losing the nipple, and even where to place the incision and how big it might be). What many people don't realize is that oftentimes achieving the best *cosmetic* result may potentially compromise achieving the best *cancer* result, and these two priorities can be in direct conflict. For example, an extremely small incision may give you a more desirable cosmetic outcome with a smaller, less noticeable scar, but a smaller incision may also make it more difficult for the surgeon to thoroughly remove all the breast tissue (which is of course the whole point of the mastectomy in the first place). Similarly, for some women, making an incision under the breast, at its very bottom, may make it difficult to reach and remove all the tissue at the very top of the breast. Instead a small central incision might be the best approach. Only your breast and plastic surgeons can look at your case, your cancer, and your particular anatomy and build and help develop the best plan. So make sure you have an experienced team that will work together to get the best *overall* outcome for you, taking into account both cure and cosmetics. Good signs to look for when making your decision about your surgical team are

1. High volume. Do the breast surgeon and the plastic surgeon each do at least fifty to one hundred breast operations per year? Many high-volume breast and plastic surgeons in big centers do hundreds more, but this is the minimum: averaging at least one to two per week.
2. A track record of working together.
3. Surgeons who work out of a top-notch institution, especially an academic medical or cancer center.
4. Knowing others who have had good results and a good experience with this team. And be wary of a team that overpromises or overemphasizes cosmetic results while downplaying the importance of the cancer operation.

reconstruction (the "plastic" part) to achieve the best possible combined result from the point of view of both cancer treatment and aesthetics. The term "oncoplastic surgery" can simply mean having reconstruction after a mastectomy. The term can also be applied to lumpectomy surgery when decision making about the incision and its orientation optimizes aesthetics, or when rearrangement of the remaining breast tissue is considered after a particularly large lumpectomy in order to fill in any gap or deficit. The truth is, most of us have been doing this all along, even before the actual phrase "oncoplastic" came into use. My advice is not to get too caught up in the hype, but there are some breast surgeons who favor this approach.

Reconstruction and insurance

Many women are concerned about payment for reconstruction—how will they afford it? They know that aesthetic plastic surgery such as face-lifts and breast augmentation can cost thousands of dollars. Thankfully, financial constraints should not be a factor if you do wish to have reconstructive surgery for breast cancer. The Women's Health and Cancer Rights Act (WHCRA), a law passed in 1998, requires all group insurance policies to cover plastic surgery related to reconstruction for breast cancer. Therefore, all women who are having a mastectomy should be offered reconstruction as part of their treatment. The law also specifically includes coverage of reconstruction of the other breast to give a more symmetrical appearance. Medicare and Medicaid cover breast reconstruction as well, so there should be no significant financial barriers for the vast majority of women.

Despite the passage of this law in 1998 and its promise of near universal coverage, however, there are still disturbing disparities. Studies have shown that lower-income women and women with lower levels of education are receiving reconstruction after mastectomy at much lower rates than higher-income women or women with higher levels of education. The women in the group who are not receiving reconstruction may simply not be aware of their options, or that the law guarantees them coverage. To start to rectify this situation, another law passed in New York State in 2010 requires hospitals and their doctors to inform breast cancer patients of the availability and coverage for reconstruction before they undergo surgery. If reconstruction services are not available at the site of treatment, patients must be informed of options elsewhere and be allowed to transfer their care to a facility that does provide reconstructive services. Other states have since followed suit, enacting similar laws mandating the provision of education and information regarding reconstruction. My hope is that the Breast Cancer Patient Education Act, introduced to Congress in 2013, will make this requirement national.

THE TAKEAWAY

- Reconstruction is an excellent option for most women who have mastectomy, and it *is* covered by insurance.
- Your team, breast surgeon and plastic surgeon working together, will help you determine the best plan for your individual case.

CHAPTER 8

Decoding Your Pathology Report

what matters and what doesn't

Much of what we need to know about a particular person's cancer is determined *after* surgery, when the pathology report comes in. During the days following surgery, the tissue that was removed is processed and examined under the microscope by a pathologist, who then writes a report describing what he or she sees in the tissue that was removed. It's the pathology report that we use to determine both the stage of the cancer and what kind of additional treatment might be needed. The problem is that most pathology reports are basically unintelligible to the layperson.

By the time I met my patient Joanna, she had already undergone her first surgery at another hospital, but because it had been discovered that she had positive margins—that is, cancer cells came up to the edge of the tissue that was removed—she required further surgery, and she had come to see me for my opinion. At this point, Joanna had been given the pathology report from her first surgery, and she was feeling extremely uncertain and confused.

"Is there a Rosetta Stone guide for speaking pathology?" Joanna asked me during our first consultation.

I told her I'd translate for her, and so she fired away: "What does moderately differentiated mean? What is Her2/neu-negative? Is my Ki67 high or low, and which is better?"

In some cases, I've sat for hours with patients dissecting every word and sentence of their report. Of course, it's only natural to want to figure out the meaning and nuance of every word in the hope of finally understanding the true nature of your disease. But the truth is that there are only a few critical things to focus on in any breast pathology report. The rest is just background noise—descriptors meaningful only as medical shorthand—that has nothing to do with your prognosis or your treatment, and which you can simply tune out.

Different hospitals and pathologists like to include different details in their pathology reports above and beyond the key factors, but most of these will not really provide any additional meaningful information. One example of an irrelevant factor that may come up in your report is your tumor's Ki67 level. While Ki67 is a measure of cell proliferation and how rapidly cells seem to be growing and dividing, it has not been proven to be a meaningful prognostic factor and has not been shown to provide important information regarding need for therapy. So if you see it in your pathology report, you don't really need to ask about it. It's not important in the big picture.

Pathology reports also tend to be very comprehensive in their description of normal findings. "Sclerosing adenosis," "fibrocystic changes," and "pseudoangiomatous stromal hyperplasia" are all a mouthful—and good luck with your pronunciation—but they are just descriptions of normal things that can be found in a healthy breast as well, and they really do not mean much in the big picture of your diagnosis and treatment.

In this chapter, we'll look at seven key elements of the pathology report that *are* important. If you see something on your pathology report and it's *not* on this list, it probably means it's not useful for determining the stage of your cancer or need for additional treatment.

THE KEY ELEMENTS OF YOUR PATHOLOGY REPORT

1. Tumor Size

Measuring tumor size primarily applies to patients with invasive cancer, not DCIS. Prior to surgery, your doctor has only been able to *estimate* your tumor size, based on what is seen on the pictures or what your surgeon feels on exam. It's not until we receive the pathology report from surgery that we can ascertain the true size of the tumor or tumors. Results from the pathology report can show a tumor that was smaller than expected, larger than expected, or about the same. In any of these instances, the tumor size is important for determining the stage of your cancer and thus your prognosis (the likely course of your disease). Even in this country, where we use the U.S. standard system of measurement, tumor size is typically measured in the metric system, as centimeters or fractions of centimeters. The average tumor size for all women diagnosed with invasive breast cancer in the United States is about 1.0 to 1.5 centimeters (around half an inch). Tumors that are smaller than a centimeter, or sub-centimeter, are usually measured in millimeters; for example, 0.5 centimeter is 5 millimeters.

> **NEED TO KNOW**
>
> If you have been diagnosed with DCIS (see chapter 5 for an explanation of DCIS), then you will most likely *not* see tumor size on your pathology report, since all DCIS, no matter how much of it you have, is considered stage 0 breast cancer. The main issue with DCIS is to make sure everything has been successfully removed—tumor size isn't a factor.

2. Margin status

For patients who have a thorough mastectomy, the entire breast is removed. With the entire breast removed, there is little remaining breast tissue and thus an extremely low possibility that cancer has been left behind. But if you have a lumpectomy, only a portion of the breast is taken, so how do we know if the entire cancer was completely re-moved? The single best indication that the cancer has been removed is a pathology report showing that the edges of the tissue removed around the cancer, or margins, are all clear (negative). The margins are the edges of the tissue surrounding the tumor, and when these edges are clear of cancer cells, we know that we have been successful in re-moving the mainstay of the cancer. When we still see cancer cells at the edges, however, the worry is that there is cancer on the other side of that edge, still in the breast. When this happens, the report comes back indicating that the margins are not clear (positive).

It's worth keeping in mind that approximately 10 to 20 percent of lumpectomy patients—up to one in five—require additional surgery to achieve clear margins. Although it may seem as if your surgeon has somehow failed you if he or she did not remove all the cancer on the first go-round, in fact a second surgery is *recognized as a potential part of the lumpectomy process* and simply means your surgeon is doing his or her job and being meticulous. Sad to say, it's almost impossible for the surgeon to accurately assess the status of the margins while surgery is being conducted (although much research is being done to address this). Cancer in the margins is microscopic and therefore impossible for the surgeon to see with the naked eye or identify through manual examination at the time of surgery.

Some people ask, "Why do I need margins that are clear if I am going to get radiation treatment afterward to deal with whatever is left behind after surgery?" This will be discussed in greater detail in the sec-tion on radiation in chapter 10, but suffice it to say that while radiation can mop up microscopic cancer cells that are left behind, it does not compensate for inadequate surgery where a significant amount of can-cer is left behind. In other words, adequate surgery involves obtaining clear margins.

No patient who is having a lumpectomy wants or hopes for a second operation, but if your pathology report does come back indicating margins that are not clear, then you will require another surgery, often referred to as a *re-excision*. Thankfully, this second surgery to remove additional tissue from the margins is usually short, is relatively low risk, and requires minimal additional recovery time. Keep in mind that your breast cancer surgery isn't complete until clear margins are achieved, and that in some cases it may even be necessary to go back in a third time to remove more tissue until the margins are fully clear. Different surgeons and institutions have different limits for the number of times they are willing to re-excise to try to get clear margins. The surgeon will also factor in your breast size and how increasingly disfigured you might become with each successive try. But for most surgeons and most patients' breasts, three times is the maximal number of attempts at getting clear margins before both you and your surgeon will start to come to terms with the fact that the cancer, on a microscopic level, is more extensive than was expected.

If after three attempts the margins are still unclear, your surgeon may recommend a mastectomy. As discussed in chapter 6, the only way to eliminate the possibility of having multiple sequential operations is to choose mastectomy, where *all* the breast tissue is removed, thereby eliminating the question of margins completely. In one uncommon scenario, the results from the first lumpectomy operation will show cancer that is surprisingly widespread. When this happens, your surgeon may recommend having a mastectomy rather than a second attempt at getting clear margins, as further surgery to get clear margins may seem unlikely to be successful.

How much tissue is enough to make a margin clear? Recent studies indicate that there is a substantial lack of agreement on what amount of tissue constitutes a clear margin. A recent consensus statement indicated that as long as the tumor cells do not come right up to the edge of the tissue removed, as though the tumor was cut through, this qualifies as clear margins. In some cases, there may be reason to want a greater margin of clearance. An experienced breast surgeon who works with an equally experienced pathologist will know how to explain margin information to you, and communicate the reasons why you do or do not need additional surgery.

3. Lymph node status

The status of the lymph nodes is the most important factor in the prognosis of women with invasive breast cancer, and also plays a significant role in determining whether and what kind of additional treatment might be necessary.

As discussed in chapter 5, women have many lymph nodes in the armpit. Although the number varies from person to person, it usually ranges from about ten to about fifty. With sentinel node biopsy, we remove only a few nodes (anywhere from one to five is most common) to examine them more closely. These nodes are then sent to the pathology laboratory, and the report will tell us whether or not cancer has spread to the nodes.

The pathology report also reveals important information about how many lymph nodes were removed and how many of these had cancer. These outcomes are frequently expressed as a fraction. For example, 0/3 means three lymph nodes were removed and none had cancer, while 2/27 means that twenty-seven lymph nodes were removed and cancer was found in two.

If sentinel nodes are normal, no further surgery is needed. If one or more nodes have cancer, then sometimes further surgery is warranted to remove the rest of the nodes. Of course no one *wants* a second operation, but we also don't want to leave behind an amount of cancer that would compromise cure. Removing the rest of the lymph nodes is called a completion axillary dissection (see chapter 5 on different types of lymph node surgery), and it's done to ensure there is no significant amount of disease left behind in the rest of the nodes. An axillary dissection is associated with a higher risk of lymphedema (also described in chapter 5), numbness, and other potential long-term side effects. An experienced breast cancer surgeon understands the complexities of the decision to go ahead with this second operation, and will be prepared to have an informed conversation with you around the risks and benefits of a subsequent surgery versus leaving the rest of the nodes alone.

What guides us in determining whether or not additional surgery is needed when positive nodes are found? Decision making can be complex, as many factors come into play. For example, we know that in many cases even when one or two sentinel lymph nodes have cancer, the rest of the nodes can safely be left alone for women who are having a lumpectomy. A recent important study called the Z11 trial showed that for women who have a lumpectomy and sentinel node biopsy where two or fewer nodes are found to have cancer, there's usually no need for subsequent surgery. Residual cancer in the rest of the nodes is unlikely, and if some does still exist, additional treatments, including radiation, will mop up any microscopic amount of disease that might be left behind. This spares many patients the larger surgery to remove the rest of the nodes. Note that it is not entirely clear yet whether *not* removing additional lymph nodes is safe for women who have a mastectomy, as most women who undergo mastectomy will *not* have radiation to follow, and thus residual microscopic cells may not get mopped up if left behind. For any patient, if three or more lymph nodes are positive or even if one or two lymph nodes are found to have a large amount of cancer in them, completion axillary dissection is often recommended.

In short, when sentinel lymph nodes are completely clear, no additional lymph node removal is warranted. When lymph nodes are involved, you and your surgeon will most likely have a discussion regarding whether additional surgery is needed. The complicated nature of this discussion—more surgery or not—is another reason to go to a breast surgery specialist, who can best guide and advise you through this complex decision making process.

4. Estrogen/progesterone receptor status

Estrogen and progesterone receptor status can usually be gleaned from a needle biopsy report. So in most situations, we already know this information prior to surgery being performed. Occasionally, if the pieces of tissue from the biopsy were very small or the amount of tumor tissue retrieved with the needle biopsy was limited, this status can only be obtained on the final pathology report after surgery. In either case, what we are looking for when we assess receptor status is whether or not the tumor's growth is being fueled by hormones. This in turn provides information about how the tumor might behave, and also provides critical information that helps us to make recommendations for treatment after surgery (see chapter 9 for more on this).

What do we mean by estrogen and progesterone receptor status? All cells, including cancer cells, have receptors that sit on the surface of the cell. I always tell patients to imagine receptors as little chairs, each with its own very particular shape. Different elements that are circulating in the blood can float by and sit down on the chair that is the perfect match for their shape and size. When the receptor chair is filled, this sends a signal into the cell telling it to trigger growth and potential spread. Estrogen and progesterone receptors on cancer cells are filled by the hormones estrogen and progesterone circulating in the body, so those hormones stimulate the cancer cells' growth. Cancers that have estrogen or progesterone receptors are called estrogen/progesterone receptor positive, or ER/PR positive, meaning that estrogen or progesterone does stimulate growth when it reaches those cells. Cancers that do not have these receptors in any amount are called estrogen/progesterone negative, or ER/PR negative, and thus hormones circulating in the body do not directly affect cancer growth or spread.

Most cancers—approximately 60 to 70 percent of those newly diagnosed—are hormone receptor positive. The main advantage of having a cancer that is estrogen or progesterone positive is that there are medications that can be given that exploit this property of the cancer, which leads to a reduction in the risk of cancer recurrence.

If your pathology report shows that your cancer is hormone receptor positive, there are a number of medications that may be prescribed for treatment. Tamoxifen is an estrogen receptor blocker, which means that it sits in the estrogen receptor chair, thereby preventing the estrogen from sitting down (picture a game of biological musical chairs). When the estrogen is blocked, the stimulus for cell growth and potential spread is blocked, thereby reducing the risk of cancer growth and spread.

Another class of drugs, called aromatase inhibitors, also works as hormonal therapy. These inhibitors function by interfering with the body's estrogen production. When estrogen production is lowered, markedly less estrogen is circulating to sit in the receptors, which means decreased chances of cancer cell growth when the cells are dependent on estrogen. Remember, these drugs that block or reduce hormones *only* work on tumors and cells that are fed by hormones (receptor-positive tumors).

5. Her2/neu status

Much like hormone receptors, Her2/neu status helps to define and characterize a tumor and what makes it grow, and also affects treatment decisions. Her2/neu is a gene that some tumors have in an excess amount. You may hear your doctor use the term "overexpress" or "amplified" to describe your Her2/neu-positivity (in other words, you have "too much" of it). Only about 10 to 20 percent of breast cancers are positive for Her2/neu. If your cancer is found to be Her2/neu-positive, then you may be given a type of targeted treatment called Herceptin that clearly reduces the risk of cancer coming back and improves survival. Additionally, Her2/neu-positivity helps predict your response to other types of chemotherapy, which in turn helps the oncologists make decisions about what type of treatment to recommend. Recently other drugs have been developed that work with Herceptin to further reduce risk of recurrence for patients with breast cancer that overexpresses Her2/neu. One, called pertuzumab (Perjeta), is often given before surgery. If you are in the minority of patients who are Her2/neu-positive, it may be beneficial to discuss the option of chemotherapy before surgery (see chapter 9 for further discussion). Herceptin and other drugs targeting Her2/neu represent some of the biggest breakthroughs in breast cancer treatment. As recently as ten years ago, before these agents were available, having a Her2/neu-positive breast cancer was an ominous sign. With these treatment agents we take an otherwise aggressive breast cancer and basically neutralize it, reducing the risk of the cancer coming back and improving survival: an important reason for optimism for this group of patients.

NEED TO KNOW

When tumors are estrogen positive, progesterone positive, Her2/neu-positive, or all three, we have targeted agents to treat them that reduce the risk of them coming back and all improve the likelihood of survival. Tumors that are estrogen negative, progesterone negative, and Her2/neu-negative are commonly referred to as "triple negative" breast cancers. Even though being Her2/neu-negative is quite common and not a bad thing, with a combined negativity of all three markers, cancers are considered more aggressive, have a higher risk of coming back, and are more difficult to treat in a targeted way (the hormonal treatments and Herceptin—all described above—don't work in these cases). However, surgical options remain the same and these cancers are certainly still curable. Approximately 10 to 15 percent of all newly diagnosed breast cancers are triple negative. But it's important to know that among African American women, triple negative cancers make up approximately 30 percent of all newly diagnosed cases, possibly contributing to the poorer overall prognosis seen in black women with breast cancer. In addition, approximately 75 percent of cancers in women with the BRCA-1 genetic predisposition are triple negative. Much current research is focusing on identifying better and more targeted treatments for triple negative breast cancer and in these specific groups of women.

A WORD TO THE WISE

For most invasive tumors, the information on estrogen, progesterone, and Her2/neu status can frequently be obtained from the needle core biopsy done to diagnose your cancer. When we have this information up front, before surgery, this can help us better direct your course of care, and will help determine if you should be seeing a medical oncologist to discuss the option of having chemotherapy *before* surgery.

6. Lymphovascular invasion

When the pathologist looks under the microscope and sees tumor cells in the small blood vessels and lymphatic channels surrounding the tumor, your pathology report will come back marked with the words "lymphovascular invasion." This does not mean that the tumor has necessarily spread; it means that tumors where cells can be seen in the surrounding blood vessels and lymphatic channels usually have more *potential* for spread than those without. There is some debate about the importance of lymphovascular invasion if the lymph nodes are negative. After all, if the tumor *can* spread (which is what lymphovascular invasion is supposed to show) but did not yet do so in any obvious way, is this factor important in and of itself? Yes, but not to the same degree. If the lymph nodes are clear and the tumor has not spread, the presence of lymphovascular invasion in and around the tumor in the breast may not affect decision making about further treatment.

7. Tumor grade

Each tumor is graded based on how aggressive the cells appear under the microscope. Grades range from grade I (or well-differentiated, meaning the least aggressive-looking) to grade III (poorly differentiated, meaning the most aggressive-looking). Most patients assume that tumor grade is extremely important in determining prognosis and further treatment, but in fact it is one of the least significant factors.

For example, we may find that a tumor is poorly differentiated, that it is small, and that the lymph nodes are normal. The fact that the tumor is grade III in and of itself will not usually impact plans for treatment; neither does it strongly affect prognosis, and it is not factored into the staging of breast cancer in any way. However, it is true that bad factors do sometimes travel in packs. For example, poorly differentiated cancers are more likely to spread to lymph nodes than well-differentiated cancers. But even a small, poorly differentiated cancer with no lymph node spread may still have a very good prognosis. In other words, while it is useful for your surgeon to know the grade of your cancer, you shouldn't obsess over a diagnosis of a "poorly differentiated" tumor, as it is only one small factor in determining your course of treatment going forward.

NEED TO KNOW

The single most important factor about prognosis—or how likely it is that you will survive your breast cancer—is lymph node status. The second most important factor is tumor size. That's why these are the two factors incorporated into the staging system. The other factors outlined above, while still meaningful and important in determining the need for additional treatment, are simply not as important as the top two in determining outcome.

CANCER STAGING: WHAT IT MEANS FOR YOU
AND HOW IT IS DETERMINED

Most patients have heard of the stages of cancer, and almost every cancer patient will be asked at some point by others, "What stage are you?" The staging of the cancer determines the extent to which the cancer has grown or spread, and it is the strongest indicator of prognosis or outcome. Formal staging of breast cancer can only be done after surgery, when we have all the results describing tumor size and analyzing the lymph nodes.

It may surprise you to learn that *only* two factors from the pathology report are involved in determining cancer stage: these are the lymph node status and tumor size. Estrogen/progesterone status, Her2/neu status, tumor grade, and the presence or absence of lymphovascular invasion are all important, but *do not* factor into the breast cancer staging system in any way. Staging for breast cancer is done using the T, N, M system, which stands for tumor size, nodal status, and metastasis. These are the pieces of information we need to determine stage.

Here are the different cancer stages and what they mean.

Stage 0: Patients who have cancer that is purely and only DCIS (see chapter 5 for a full explanation of DCIS) are stage 0. Regardless of the *amount* of DCIS present in the breast—whether involving a small part or the whole breast—when no invasive cancer is present, the stage is considered 0.

Stage 1: When even the most minuscule amount of invasive cancer has broken through the breast duct, this pushes a woman into stage 1. Stage 1 is defined as tumors smaller than two centimeters (a little under an inch) with normal lymph nodes found at surgery.

Stage 2: When tumors are larger than two centimeters or lymph nodes are involved, breast cancer has reached stage 2.

Stage 3: The difference between stage 2 and stage 3 is defined by larger tumors and more extensive lymph node involvement. Stage 3 includes tumors that are more advanced, with invasion into the underlying pec muscle or overlying skin. Stage 3 also includes inflammatory breast cancer, categorized as stage 3B (see chapter 5 for an explanation of inflammatory cancer). With positive lymph nodes above the collarbone or clavicle, breast cancer is categorized as stage 3C. It also includes cases with positive lymph nodes inside the breastbone or sternum, called internal mammary nodes. These lymph nodes are generally detected on physical examination of the neck or scans of the body done in advanced cases. These nodes are generally not removable through surgery, as their locations make them difficult to reach safely, but chemotherapy and radiation can eradicate them. (For more on different lymph node basins, see chapter 5 in the section on lymph nodes.)

Stage 4: Breast cancer that has spread to other parts of the body. People with breast cancer at stages 0 to 3 are *all* curable, and treatment can be undertaken with intent to cure. When breast cancer has spread to other parts of the body—commonly the lungs, liver, bone, and brain—the disease is still treatable, but in general it is no longer considered curable. Patients can live for years with treatment for stage 4 disease, but even for patients who seem to be in remission, the cancer will usually come back, because circulating cells can almost never be completely and permanently eradicated.

For patients who are found to have stage 4 disease at the time of first diagnosis, the role of surgery is very controversial. By now, the disease has already spread and many people question whether removing the main tumor and/or lymph nodes provides any benefit if there is still cancer left elsewhere in the body. Some feel that removing the main tumor prevents further seeding of tumor cells and spread, thereby helping to control disease. Others theorize that the main tumor might actually hold the spread in check, and therefore removing it might lead to an explosive growth of tumors elsewhere and further spread. Much research is being devoted to answering the question of whether or not to remove a tumor when the patient has stage 4 breast cancer. If you are diagnosed with stage 4 disease, therefore, decisions about surgery need to be made on a case-by-case basis, with access to the very latest research, and with true specialists at a top-notch center guiding you.

Some women, particularly those who undergo a mastectomy, may have more than one individual tumor in the breast. It's important to know that to determine your stage when there are multiple tumors, we use the tumor size of the *largest* individual tumor; we don't add them all together. So, for example, if you have three separate tumors within the breast that are 1.5, 1.0, and 0.5 centimeters and normal lymph nodes, for staging purposes your cancer is 1.5 cm (not the sum total of 3.0 centimeters) and thus stage 1.

THE TAKEAWAY

- Tumor size and lymph nodes status are the factors that determine cancer stage and are most important when it comes to prognosis.
- Margin status is an important factor in lumpectomy surgery to make sure you have the best chance that the cancer has been effectively removed, and thus the lowest risk of cancer recurrence in the breast.
- The other pathology report descriptors factor into prognosis and decision making about further treatment.

CHAPTER 9

Chemo, Medication, and All the Options

when you need to see a medical oncologist

Once the pathology report is available and you have reviewed it with your surgeon—who has determined that you don't need any more surgery—the next step is usually to determine if you need additional treatment. Additional treatments, such as medicine or radiation, are also sometimes referred to as *adjuvant* treatments, because they are added on to surgery. Usually the first doctor you will see after surgery is a medical oncologist. As the name suggests, a medical oncologist is someone who gives medicine to reduce the risk of the cancer coming back. These medicines include chemotherapy (usually given intravenously) and hormonal therapy, also called endocrine therapy (usually given in pill form). Some women get both chemotherapy and hormonal drugs, while some women need nothing additional, as surgery alone is enough. As with everything in breast cancer, there is no one-size-fits-all approach. If you have a friend who needed chemotherapy after surgery, this does not necessarily mean that you will too, even if you and she seem to have similar stages and situations. There are cases where chemotherapy is given first, even before surgery, to shrink the tumor; more on this will follow.

For this next stage of your treatment, I highly recommend that you seek out an oncologist who focuses exclusively or primarily on breast cancer. The options for treatment are expanding and improving every year, so you need to work with someone who is up to date on the latest. When you choose to receive your care in a specialized breast center or major medical center, often the breast surgeon will be able to refer you directly to the medical oncologist within the same facility. This model of seamless, coordinated care is often comforting, given that logistical issues, such as making appointments and transferring records, are often taken care of for you. But you may also choose to have different aspects of care in different facilities based on factors such as referrals from other doctors, reputation, and recommendations from fellow patients. And while it's never advisable to pick a doctor *solely* based on convenience, proximity can factor in when it comes to selecting your medical oncologist, given that chemotherapy usually involves a series of treatments stretched over a longer period of time. As noted before, it's important for your oncologist to specialize in breast cancer, with a significant portion of his or her practice devoted to taking care of breast cancer patients. Confirm that your oncologist did accredited fellowship training in oncology, preferably in a well-recognized academic medical center. And many breast medical oncologists did additional years of training focusing solely on breast cancer.

A WORD TO THE WISE

With surgery, there are two major parts of the surgeon's role: the decision making and the doing. Two surgeons may both decide that you need a mastectomy, but they may do the actual operation differently. With medical oncology, it is almost all about decision making and not about the doing. Once it is decided that your plan is to receive a specific treatment, getting that specific drug or medication can happen almost anywhere, as the actual delivery of the medication does not vary significantly from place to place and from oncologist to oncologist. There are definitely some potential benefits to being treated at a major medical center, including the availability of some special, institution-specific protocols or cutting-edge trials. In addition, medical oncologists at specialized centers often have their fingers on the pulse of the newest developments and the best options for treatment in each different scenario, and may have more experience in dealing with complications related to treatment. But if you prefer to be treated locally and there is no specialized oncologist, often the best strategy is to travel to at least get an opinion from a specialized breast medical oncologist at a reputable center who can help you decide on the best treatment plan. Then, if there is nothing specific to your case that can benefit from being treated at a particular institution and the regimen recommended is standard (which is the case for most women), you can actually then feel confident in receiving the same treatment closer to home.

When further treatment *is* needed

After my patient Susan was diagnosed, her surgery revealed that the cancer had spread to her lymph nodes and that a total of three of her twenty-one lymph nodes removed were cancerous. In Susan's case both chemotherapy *and* endocrine therapy were recommended, which is quite common for women with cancer that has spread to the lymph nodes.

Like so many of my patients, Susan wanted to know more. "If the cancer was removed with surgery, why would I need additional treatment?" she asked.

I explained to Susan that her cancer had already grown over the course of months and even years before it was found. What started out as one bad cell divided into two bad cells. Two bad cells divided into four bad cells. This process of cells growing and dividing had continued until, by the time her cancer was just a centimeter (less than half an inch), there were about a billion bad cells. Some of these cells traveled to her lymph nodes, which is why three nodes with cancer were found and removed. When positive lymph nodes are found, it means that there is a higher chance that cancer cells could have taken the next step as well: escaping into the body, circulating in the bloodstream, and waiting to take up residence somewhere else, or metastasizing. If those cells *did* metastasize, her breast cancer would become incurable. I explained to Susan that even though she had scans of the body that thankfully were normal, these scans had limitations and could only show obvious spread, not microscopic spread. This possibility of microscopic cell escape in patients with newly diagnosed breast cancer is the reason additional medical treatment is given, and why we need medical oncologists.

Fortunately, we have many effective options for treatment, both in terms of chemotherapy and medicine, with more being developed every year through excellent research efforts. When combined with surgery, these treatments can provide excellent outcomes and prognosis for most, giving all of us reasons to be optimistic.

How doctors determine the need for further treatment

Most surgeons will tell their patients after surgery if they need to meet with a medical oncologist to discuss potential further aspects of their care, and most women with breast cancer will need to meet with this specialist. When you meet with your medical oncologist, he or she is going to discuss the options and recommendations regarding your additional treatment. The medical oncologist's job is to take the information obtained from surgery—as described in the pathology report—and to use this information to determine what the approximate risk is of microscopic spread. Your doctor will then combine this information on risk of spread with information about your *individual* case. Factors such as your age, underlying medical conditions, and overall health are taken into account before coming up with a recommendation for the best treatment plan. If the risk of spread is low, then additional treatment may be of little added benefit. For example, patients with DCIS have almost no risk of spread (see chapter 5 for an explanation of DCIS), so the added benefit of chemotherapy is close to zero and is never given. If you have invasive cancer and the risk of spread in your particular case is higher, then treatment of some sort will most likely be recommended. Then there are the patients who fall somewhere in the middle. More on that to come.

Options for treatment

In general, treatment falls into two main categories: chemotherapy, which is usually given intravenously, and hormonal or endocrine therapy, which is usually in pill form. So for any given patient there will be four possible courses of treatment:

1. Chemotherapy alone
2. Hormonal therapy alone
3. Both
4. Neither.

Chemotherapy: what to expect

Chemotherapy is a category of cancer treatment that uses strong chemical medicines, usually given through an IV so that they can circulate in the bloodstream killing any microscopic cancer cells that may have escaped into the body. Treatment is usually given in a chemotherapy center on an outpatient basis and is dripped through the IV fairly slowly; the total time for treatment can take a few hours per session. Most chemotherapy is given in cycles extending over a period of months, with the goal of giving the body and its normal cells enough time to recover between treatments. The standard treatment regimens typically involve one treatment cycle every two or three weeks for six or eight treatments. As a result, chemotherapy can last anywhere from four to six months.

Many women understandably fear the side effects of chemotherapy. We've all seen the images of hair loss on TV or in the movies, and seen depictions of women running to the bathroom to vomit every few minutes. As with many things, the Hollywood version of chemotherapy does not really provide a good representation of the real thing. While chemotherapy *does* have side effects, the side effects differ by regimen, they are usually tolerable, and the worst aspects are short-term. For some women, finding out that they need chemotherapy crushes their hope of keeping their diagnosis of breast cancer private: while they may have been able to go through surgery, especially a lumpectomy, without widely sharing with others, losing one's hair (a side effect from some chemo treatments, but not all) is harder (but not impossible) to hide.

How your oncologist will determine the need for chemotherapy

The main factors that will help your oncologist determine the need for chemotherapy are lymph node status, tumor size, and the tumor profile (estrogen, progesterone, and Her2/neu; see chapter 8). If you've been found to have positive lymph nodes, it's usually recommended that you have chemotherapy, since a tumor that has spread to the lymph nodes has shown that it has a higher capacity for traveling, and ultimately for spreading to other parts of the body. The likelihood of spread beyond the lymph nodes is directly related to the amount of lymph node involvement. So having one lymph node involved is probably better than having three lymph nodes involved, which is better than having ten lymph nodes involved.

While lymph node involvement is certainly the most important factor in determining the need for chemotherapy, treatment is also recommended for many patients even when lymph nodes are not involved. There is no absolute tumor size cutoff that determines that you will or will not get chemotherapy, but if the tumor is large enough, chemotherapy may be recommended based on this criterion as well. As a general rule, for younger, premenopausal patients with tumors larger than a centimeter (and even some with tumors smaller than that), chemotherapy will at least be considered. It follows that for many patients with very small tumor sizes and negative lymph nodes, the likelihood of spread is so low that the risks of chemotherapy and the potential side effects outweigh its benefits and chemotherapy is often not recommended.

Estrogen and progesterone status as well as Her2/neu status (see chapter 8 for full discussions of these) also factor in heavily and influence decision making. Her2/neu-positive tumors are very responsive to certain types of chemotherapy, and specific targeted therapy is also quite effective and therefore usually given. Some type of treatment will be recommended for almost all women whose tumors are Her2/neu-positive, unless the tumor was quite small with normal nodes.

Women whose tumors are estrogen and progesterone receptor negative or "triple negative" also usually require chemotherapy, again unless the tumor was quite small and lymph nodes are normal.

A WORD TO THE WISE

Everyone wants definitive answers about her disease and prognosis. As you speak with your medical oncologist about your ongoing treatment, however, you need to keep in mind that there is no test or definitive way of assessing risk for cancer spread after surgery. As doctors, we can only estimate. If there was a blood test or scan that could tell us who has microscopic spread and who doesn't, we would know for certain who needs chemotherapy and who doesn't. There is much research being directed toward developing this sort of test, but because no such test currently exists, doctors recommend chemotherapy for many patients as a precaution, without actually knowing whether it will or will not benefit them.

It's also important to understand that chemotherapy does not work in every case. If it did, then every patient would have surgery and then chemotherapy and the cancer would be cured for sure, forever. The fact remains that patients who have had surgery and chemotherapy can still develop metastatic disease (where microscopic cells have spread and chemotherapy didn't work against them). But cure rates for breast cancer, all types, have never been better because fortunately, in most cases, the combination of treatments *does* work.

Often the choice lies with you

There are many patients who fall in between the clear-cut high- and low-risk categories, with a risk of microscopic spread somewhere in the middle, and you may find yourself in this situation. As a result, you often have a choice of whether to move forward with chemotherapy or not. In the same way that the breast surgeon will guide you through the complex decision-making process around lumpectomy versus mastectomy, a trusted medical oncologist will do the same when it comes to additional treatment. He or she will weigh many different factors about your cancer (tumor size, lymph node status, hormone receptor status, Her2/neu status, and other factors), then combine this information with factors about you (age, overall health, and of course your preference). Only then can he or she help guide you toward the right decision for you regarding taking additional treatment. And just like deciding between lumpectomy and mastectomy, making a decision about additional treatment can be straightforward or it can be complicated, depending on your case and your preferences. This is why you really need a specialized breast medical oncologist to lead you through the process, so you can feel confident that you are on the right path.

Chemotherapy regimens

Different types of chemotherapy regimens work for different types of tumors. We don't give the same kind of chemotherapy to people with breast cancer as we give to people with colon cancer. There are even different options for chemotherapy treatment for patients *within* the breast cancer category. Sometimes only one chemotherapy medicine is given, but more often a few different agents are combined into a single regimen. Each chemotherapy regimen and type of medicine given has its own set of side effects, some mild, some stronger. So the medical oncologist's goal is to take all these variables into account and recommend the right treatment regimen for *you*. The good news is that newer, better chemotherapeutic agents are being developed all the time to help further improve survival while reducing side effects.

The side effects

Everyone knows that chemotherapy comes with side effects, but it's important to know that every woman will experience chemotherapy differently. Chemotherapy can be a walk in the park for some women; for others, it's brutal and incapacitating. If you have been told that you need chemotherapy and you are nervous about side effects, my advice is to remember that for the most part the side effects are temporary. In general, the good cells recover, while hopefully cancer cells do not.

- **Hair loss.** For many women, hair loss, while not a major medical side effect, is a primary concern because of the profound effect it can have on appearance and self-image. This is one of the only side effects that you wear on the outside, making your disease evident to the rest of the world. Many moms are concerned about the dramatic effect their hair loss might have on their children, making them appear clearly different and even sick. (See chapter 3 for tips on how to talk to your children about breast cancer.) For sure it can be a tough process to lose your hair, but there are some well-made and very natural-looking wigs out there that can do a great job of disguising hair loss. The key is to remember it's a temporary state, and that your hair will always grow back over time. It may grow back slightly differently from before: women with previously straight hair might notice some curliness, especially when it's still short. And if you previously colored your hair, of course it won't naturally grow back the same shade that you got from a bottle before it fell out. But in time you will be able to color and style it however you want.

  If hair loss is your single most dreaded side effect related to chemotherapy, you might want to know about a relatively new development called the cold cap. The cold cap looks like a space age bathing cap that is worn during chemotherapy. The cap is connected to a machine that circulates icy cold water through the cap, thus slowing blood flow to the scalp and the hair follicles. With slower blood flow to this part of the body, chemotherapy (which circulates in the bloodstream during delivery) does not reach the hair follicles and usually results in preservation of hair for the duration of chemotherapy treatment. The cold cap has been used for years now in Europe and is slowly gaining traction in the United States. Its increasing popularity is understandable given that for many women, hair loss not only affects how they look and feel, but is also the only factor that jeopardizes their chance to keep their cancer diagnosis and treatment private. And I think it is safe to say that if given the choice, no woman would actually elect to lose her hair if she didn't have to.

  But if the cold cap had no downsides everyone would do it, right? Here are the disadvantages: 1) Wearing the cold cap can be intolerable for some. Some of my patients who have used it describe it as the worst eating-an-ice-cream-too-fast-headache they have ever had. That lasted for four hours. The discomfort bordering on pain has been simply too much for some to follow through and reap the benefit. 2) Hair preservation may not work for all women, so you can endure the experience and end up with only clumps of hair preserved; not an ideal result. 3) It's important to know that currently, it is *not* FDA approved, and is not currently reimbursable by insurance, which brings me to number 4) The cold cap is expensive. The cap and the machine that it is connected to are run by companies that charge for the service and the sessions. It can thus run in excess of thousands of dollars to complete all the necessary chemotherapy treatments with the cold cap in place. And lastly, and perhaps most important, some oncologists feel that the cold cap has not been adequately tested in randomized trials to know for sure that it won't compromise survival. The concern is that having a "no-flow" zone for chemotherapy may create a potential reservoir for cancer cells to live and hide out. If chemotherapy does not reach cancer cells, it can't eradicate them, potentially leaving them to resume circulation. Skeptics also raise the concern that if chemotherapy doesn't reach a part of the body (the scalp), perhaps that part of the body is at higher risk for developing metastasis in the future. This is mostly a theoretical risk, as many European studies using the cold cap have not shown a higher incidence of scalp metastasis, a very rare occurrence in any case. Most oncologists will currently only feel comfortable even considering use of the cold cap in cases where cancer is not very advanced, and the cap is not a real potential risk of compromising care in any way.

- **Nausea.** Everyone has experienced nausea at some point or another and knows how unpleasant the sensation can be. Many women won't experience nausea at all, but if you do feel sick, there are many medications to help control it. The timing of the nausea is often related closely to when the treatment is given, and thus preemptive strikes can be made with medication to reduce the severity. So talk to your oncologist if nausea is a major side effect for you.

- **Low blood counts.** As chemotherapy goes to work on bad cells, good cells can also be affected, and blood cells, both red and white, are particularly vulnerable to these effects. Reduced red cell count can lead to anemia and fatigue, and reduced white cell count can lead to a suppressed immune system and vulnerability to infection. Signs of infection, such as fever, flulike symptoms, and coughing, need to be monitored closely, and occasionally a woman will need to be treated with antibiotics or even admitted to the hospital for treatment. Medications are available and frequently given to support cell production and prevent counts from going too low, and these are given routinely with some chemotherapy regimens. "Dose-dense" chemotherapy, which is chemotherapy given every two weeks, does not give normal cells as much time to recover, and thus medications to stimulate white cell production, such as Neupogen, are often routinely given as part of this plan.
- **Neuropathy.** One agent commonly given to breast cancer patients, Taxol, comes with an increased risk of neuropathy, meaning problems related to the nerves, including pain, numbness and tingling, or weakness, particularly in the hands and feet. Sometimes this side effect is temporary; however, some patients are left with residual deficits. If you start to experience neuropathy, often the dose of chemotherapy can be reduced or treatments changed to reduce long-term effects.
- **Appetite and taste changes.** With certain types of chemotherapy, you may experience an unpleasant metallic taste in your mouth, and appetite can definitely be affected as well. Sometimes patients report that they have a decreased appetite and sometimes an increased one. Often steroids are given to control side effects related to chemotherapy, and these can affect appetite and even lead to cravings for things like carbs and comfort foods. So the notion that chemotherapy inevitably leads to weight loss can actually be a misconception. And weight *gain* during chemotherapy—to the chagrin of many women—is actually quite common and can add insult to injury, especially if a woman was already struggling to control her weight going in to her treatment. I appreciate this, and I hate that, above all else she is dealing with, my

patient might be additionally concerned about weight gain. But I urge all my patients to do their best, not get too down on themselves, and understand it's not realistic to try to deal with too many things at once. After chemotherapy is over, when your energy increases and recovery is well under way, is the time to address any concerns regarding weight.

- **Mouth sores.** Some chemotherapy causes mouth sores, and many oncologists offer their patients ice chips, which reduce blood flow and thus chemotherapy flow to the tongue and mouth, to reduce this.

- **Constipation and diarrhea.** Bowel habits can be affected by chemotherapy, both because of chemo's effects on diet changes and appetite and for other reasons. Although diarrhea and constipation can develop, these issues are rarely serious, and medication to address either of them is definitely available and effective.

- **"Chemo-brain."** Many patients find that during chemotherapy, they feel foggy and tend to be more forgetful. Thankfully, chemotherapy is not associated with a likelihood of long-term cognitive deficits. Although some patients describe these effects as long-lasting, for most women there is full recovery after treatment. Many of my most intelligent (and self-deprecating) patients joke that now they have a better excuse for forgetting stuff that they never remembered anyway. It's important to remember that cognition and brain function can also be affected by many other factors related to breast cancer treatment outside of chemotherapy. These factors include anxiety, sleep disturbances, stress, other medications, and mood changes (such as depression). So if you are concerned about changes in your cognitive function, it is certainly worth a discussion with your medical oncologist and a deeper look at potential causes, most of which can be proactively addressed. Many breast centers and major medical and cancer centers have neurology programs that specifically test for and assess cognitive changes related to chemotherapy treatment. They can also monitor for changes using serial examinations and assessments, and many have programs and interventions (such as mind and memory exercises and routines) that can be suggested and implemented.

- **Menopause.** Menopausal-type side effects and even bringing on actual menopause are potential side effects of chemotherapy. The likelihood of going through menopause is directly related to how close you are to menopausal age at the time of treatment and the agents used in your chemotherapy regimen.
- **Other cancers.** One commonly used type of chemotherapy, cyclophosphamide (also known as Cytoxan), is associated with a higher risk of developing leukemia in the future. The increased risk of leukemia with chemotherapy compared to women who have not received chemotherapy is extremely low, approximately 1 percent. But even though the risk is low, it's still important to consider because getting leukemia is such a serious side effect, and can be life-threatening itself. And it should definitely be taken into account in your decision making if it's not certain that you need treatment.

Coping with the emotional fallout of chemotherapy

While all women have some trepidation about proceeding with chemotherapy, many are actually eager for the treatment to begin, thinking of it as further protection against cancer coming back. And as hard as it can be to undergo chemo, I've known patients who actually feel nervous when chemotherapy ends, as if a layer of protection against the cancer has gone away. In other words, whether you're about to begin chemo, are going through the treatment, or have come out the other end, your emotional reaction can be intense and surprisingly complex.

Unlike surgery, where you can gear up for a single event that is quickly completed, chemotherapy is more of a marathon than a sprint. Treatments can be given over the course of four to six months, and during that time there's no doubt that you will experience a range of emotions. Stronger feelings that interfere with coping and recovery, such as depression and hopelessness, can develop as well, and most good breast centers have many resources to support you: everything from support groups to private therapy to medication can be helpful, in both the short and long terms. I make sure that my patients understand that many women experience these feelings, that there is help available if they need it, and that seeking help is a sign of strength, not weakness.

MYTH: "You don't need chemo. Your body can fight the cancer on its own."

You may have heard stories of people who declined chemotherapy and are doing absolutely fine. When someone—usually a celebrity or self-proclaimed "expert"—starts advising others that they don't need standard treatment, keep in mind that this person may be describing his or her individual experience of getting lucky. It's true, not everyone needs chemotherapy, but until we have a reliable way of distinguishing who does need chemo from who doesn't, we often err on the side of giving treatment if there is some appreciable chance of recurrence, to reduce that risk. So my advice is to listen to your doctor, who will give you the actual information on the potential risks and benefits of the treatment being recommended for your particular case, and tune out the noise of other sources trying to throw in their two cents about their own choices, which probably have nothing to do with you and your case.

If you think about it, you're unlikely to hear from the person who refused treatment and ended up paying the price. When the cancer comes back, no one wants to admit that her own choices and actions may have contributed to a bad outcome. The people who shout to the world that they beat cancer by doing it their own way would never write a book admitting their regrets about not taking the treatment when the cancer came back.

A WORD TO THE WISE

For women who develop breast cancer at a young age, chemotherapy can put you into early menopause. So if there is the possibility that you may want to have children in the future, it is important to look into fertility preservation options *before* initiating chemotherapy (see chapter 17 for a full discussion on breast cancer and pregnancy). Many top-notch breast centers have well-established oncofertility programs in which a fertility specialist will coordinate care with your oncologists to determine timing and safety of egg or embryo harvest and preservation prior to the initiation of chemotherapy. This collaboration between fertility specialist, surgeon, and oncologist will ideally optimize your chances for successful pregnancy after treatment with the least amount of disruption or compromise to your cancer care.

Hormonal treatment

When a breast cancer is shown to be estrogen or progesterone receptor positive—which includes approximately 60 to 70 percent of all newly diagnosed cases—hormonal or endocrine treatment is usually part of the plan (for a full description of receptors and hormones go to chapter 8). The most commonly given hormonal medications are tamoxifen and the drugs called aromatase inhibitors (AIs). Both tamoxifen and AIs are recommended as further treatment after surgery for most women with hormone-positive breast cancers, and effectively reduce the risk of cancer coming back by 40 to 50 percent. So, as an example, if you are a woman with an estrogen-positive cancer that is associated with a 90 percent chance of survival (or, said differently, a 10 percent chance of recurrence), taking tamoxifen would increase your chances of survival to 95 percent. Tamoxifen has been around for more than forty years and is still one of the most effective medications for treating hormone-positive breast cancer.

For women with invasive breast cancer that is receptor-positive, hormonal treatment has three major benefits. And because the duration of treatment is years, these benefits are ongoing and long-term— another reason for optimism:

1. Hormonal treatment reduces the risk of cancer metastasizing by killing tumor cells that may be circulating.
2. It reduces the risk of cancer coming back in the same breast (for women who have had a lumpectomy).
3. It reduces the risk of developing a new cancer in the opposite breast.

Hormonal or endocrine therapy is usually taken as a pill, so it's easier than chemo. Usually patients take one pill a day, and treatment usually lasts for five to ten years. There is one less commonly used endocrine therapy agent, called Faslodex, which is given as an injection. If needed, your medical oncologist will prescribe these drugs based on your age, medical history, and menopausal status.

If you're postmenopausal: Both tamoxifen and AIs work in postmenopausal women, but major studies show that AIs work better than tamoxifen for most women in this category. As a result, AIs are now usually the drugs of choice for postmenopausal women with ER-positive cancers.

If you're premenopausal: For premenopausal women, AIs are *not* effective, and thus tamoxifen is currently still the only choice. So if you are premenopausal with an ER-positive tumor, tamoxifen will most likely be recommended. Recent studies have shown that in some cases of high risk breast cancer in premenopausal women, rendering them menopausal (usually with medication that suppresses ovarian function), and then giving them an AI might lead to even lower risks of recurrence than with tamoxifen, and so this path might be discussed with your oncologist as well.

If you have DCIS only: While chemotherapy is *only* given for patients with invasive cancer, hormonal therapy can be given for both invasive cancer and DCIS. While hormonal therapy improves survival for women with invasive cancer, for women with DCIS, survival is so high already, 98–99 percent, that neither chemotherapy nor hormonal therapy provides much added value in this arena. However, for women with DCIS, hormonal therapy is still often given for the other two benefits of reducing the risk of recurrence in the same breast for women who have had a lumpectomy, and reducing the risk of developing a new cancer in the other breast.

If you have DCIS and had a mastectomy: Women with DCIS who have had a mastectomy not only have little risk of spread but also have very little risk of recurrence in that removed breast, so the added benefit of hormonal treatment is only to reduce the already small risk of developing a new cancer on the other side. For this benefit alone, tamoxifen or AIs are usually *not* given after a mastectomy for DCIS.

If you have receptor-negative cancer: If your tumor is estrogen and progesterone receptor negative, endocrine therapy serves no purpose, since hormones were not stimulating tumor growth in the first place. So for patients with receptor-negative tumors, as they are called, the only treatment that we offer is chemotherapy.

Length of treatment

Much research has been done to determine the optimal length of time for tamoxifen and AI treatment, balancing the benefits of improved survival with the risk of side effects (see below). For many years, the optimal length of treatment with tamoxifen was thought to be five years, based on combined data from numerous studies involving thousands of patients. In 2013, however, the results from a game-changing study showed that for most premenopausal women, taking tamoxifen for ten years leads to even further reduction in cancer recurrence. Thus recommendations for length of treatment were recently changed to ten years for most premenopausal women. For some women this was welcome news: their daily tamoxifen pill provided a sense of actively extending treatment and further protection against cancer recurrence. For others who experience unpleasant side effects and are anxious to finish treatment, the decision to extend treatment is a mixed blessing. A dedicated breast medical oncologist will discuss the pros and cons of different lengths of treatment in your particular case.

The side effects

Tamoxifen is a medication that has been around since the 1970s. It has been extensively studied, and what we have seen is that for most women taking tamoxifen, the likelihood of developing *serious* side effects is extremely rare, especially when compared to the significant benefit of lowering the risk of breast cancer recurrence. Women who take tamoxifen can sometimes experience menopausal-like symptoms, including hot flashes and vaginal dryness or discharge. They also have a slightly higher risk of developing blood clots (similar to the risk associated with birth control pills), and while tamoxifen is not thought to *cause* cataracts, if you already have them tamoxifen may make them worse, and thus you may need to be monitored more closely. Perhaps the most notorious of tamoxifen's side effects is that it is associated with a minimally higher risk of developing uterine cancer, mainly in postmenopausal women. I hear many women ask, "Why would I want to take a medicine like tamoxifen to treat one cancer [of the breast] if a potential side effect is that it might cause another cancer [of the uterus]?" It's important to know that tamoxifen is primarily recommended to premenopausal women now that aromatase inhibitors are the drug of choice in postmenopausal women. And in premenopausal women, most studies have shown that tamoxifen is not associated with a substantial increased risk of uterine cancer.

MYTH: "If you are on tamoxifen for breast cancer prevention or treatment, you should be regularly checked and screened by your gynecologist for uterine cancer."

In fact, for women on tamoxifen, the risk of uterine cancer is very low, and almost all cases of uterine cancer can be detected at their earliest stage without any special screening tests, since the first warning sign is usually abnormal vaginal bleeding or spotting. All women who are on tamoxifen who have not previously had their uterus removed (a hysterectomy) should be counseled to immediately report any signs of irregular or abnormally heavy vaginal bleeding or spotting during or between menstrual periods. Because uterine cancer is picked up so early with this warning sign alone, the general recommendations from most oncology and gynecology organizations and societies is *not* to perform unnecessary additional screening exams, such as pelvic ultrasounds, with the goal of detecting uterine cancer. These exams will usually lead to false positive findings and potentially many unnecessary subsequent tests such as D&Cs, uterine biopsies, and many follow-up exams. So in summary, if your medical oncologist recommends tamoxifen, don't decline to take it based on the misconception that there is a high risk of associated and serious side effects. For most women with breast cancer, the strong benefits of reduction in breast cancer recurrence outweigh the small risks of serious medical side effects by far, and in general, aggressive screening for uterine cancer is not recommended.

For AIs, the main side effects are hot flashes, and bone and joint issues including thinning of the bones and bone and joint pain. Many women on AIs need bone density monitoring to make sure they are not developing osteoporosis.

NEED TO KNOW

Because tamoxifen is given primarily to premenopausal women—which includes women of childbearing age—it's important to know that even if your period stops, you *can* become pregnant while on tamoxifen, but should never do so. The reason? Tamoxifen can cause significant birth defects. So have a serious talk with your gynecologist, breast cancer surgeon, or oncologist about how to safely and reliably prevent pregnancy while on tamoxifen. And if getting pregnant *is* a priority, discussing the risks and benefits of stopping tamoxifen is important too. (See chapter 17 on pregnancy after breast cancer.)

When you need chemotherapy *and* hormonal therapy

Some women need both chemotherapy and endocrine therapy. For example, a premenopausal woman who has positive lymph nodes and is also hormone receptor positive will receive a course of chemotherapy and will be advised to take tamoxifen subsequently, for either five or ten years. For patients who do need both, these treatments are given sequentially, not concurrently, with chemotherapy almost always given first, followed by the hormonal treatment. For women who will have chemotherapy and hormonal therapy and also need radiation as part of their treatment regimen, treatment is still given sequentially, with the most common order of treatment being surgery first, chemotherapy second, radiation third, and the lengthy five- to ten-year hormonal treatment last, starting only after radiation is completed. The reason for sequential treatment is that some treatments may actually compete with each other, and giving one type of treatment at a time is felt to maximize the benefit of each.

Tumor profiling: another step forward in personalizing decision making for chemotherapy

For many patients the decision to undergo or forgo chemotherapy is complicated by the fact that we do not know a lot about the biologic behavior and aggressiveness of any individual cancer. In most cases, we can't know for certain whether chemotherapy is truly going to make a difference. Of course we know that in general, spread to the lymph nodes and larger tumor size increase the likelihood that the tumor is more aggressive and has spread, but these are crude measures at best. Some tumors may percolate along locally for years without any threat of spread, while others seemingly pop up out of nowhere, even immediately after a normal-appearing mammogram.

In the last ten years, however, some significant steps have been made toward personalizing decision making around whether or not to have chemotherapy. Our biggest leap forward is that we can now look at a genetic profile of an individual's tumor, which can help us determine whether there is a greater or lesser need for and potential benefit from further treatment. There are a few of these commercially available tests now available and commonly used. One, the Oncotype DX assay, can currently be performed *only* on estrogen-receptor-positive tumors, and mainly for tumors that have not spread to the lymph nodes.

With tumor profiling assays, a piece of the tumor from what was removed at surgery is sent away to a lab to be tested, and after a number of key genes in the tumor are analyzed, the results come back showing whether the tumor is at a low, intermediate, or high risk of recurrence. In some cases, patients with small tumors who would not ordinarily be recommended to have chemotherapy are found to have surprisingly aggressive cancers based on their genetic profile, and chemotherapy is given. More often, a patient who ordinarily would have received chemotherapy based on having a slightly larger tumor is found to have a low or intermediate recurrence score, and the option to forgo chemotherapy is now reasonable. Oncotype testing has become an essential tool for medical oncologists to help guide their patients, and it has taken personalized decision making for adjuvant treatment to the next level. It has also added another level of complexity to decision making regarding treatment for women with ER-positive tumors. This complexity and the level of expertise necessary to understand it is another reason you should seek out a specialized breast medical oncologist for your care. And if your tumor fits into the ER-positive, node-negative category and oncotype testing has not been requested, by all means ask why not.

Some research has also been done and is currently ongoing to try to expand the use and role of oncotype testing by studying its relevance in patients with positive nodes, as well as other clinical scenarios, so we can better pick and choose those who should receive and are more likely to benefit from chemotherapy. For example, just because a patient has a positive node does not necessarily mean that the cancer has spread beyond that. If it hasn't, then certainly chemotherapy would not be of any added value. While no test at this time will give us that information definitively, oncotype testing in this group could be an indicator. There are other commercially available similar genetic profiling tests, such as the Mammaprint, and others are on the way that may provide us with even more precision when it comes to making decisions about adjuvant treatment.

Neoadjuvant chemotherapy: when chemotherapy is given first

For most patients, surgery comes first and then additional treatments such as chemotherapy come after. Studies have shown that there is no real survival advantage associated with the order of treatment (chemotherapy first, surgery after versus surgery first, chemo after), and so we usually perform surgery first because we know we can obtain important information from the pathology report to help guide treatment down the line. However, in some cases, doing chemotherapy first does provide some benefit. When chemotherapy comes first, we call this *neoadjuvant* chemotherapy.

Neoadjuvant chemotherapy is usually recommended in the following cases:

1. For patients with inflammatory breast cancer, neoadjuvant chemotherapy is always done first (see chapter 5 for an explanation of inflammatory cancer). Without chemotherapy to shrink the cancer, the area involved would be much too extensive to successfully remove everything with surgery.

2. In some cases the tumor is too large, is attached to the chest wall, or involves the overlying skin in a way that makes surgery, even a mastectomy, difficult or impossible to perform successfully. In these cases, it is often recommended to give chemotherapy first, again to shrink the tumor and facilitate a better outcome with surgery afterward.

3. Neoadjuvant chemotherapy is sometimes recommended for tumors that are borderline in size for a lumpectomy, where shrinking them down even a bit might optimize the chances of successfully performing a lumpectomy for patients who are motivated to have a smaller surgery and try to save their breast.

4. Patients with triple negative cancers (negative for estrogen, progesterone, and Her2/neu) and those that are Her2/neu-positive are also often advised to have chemotherapy before surgery. These patients have tumors that are known to respond best and most exuberantly to chemotherapy, and thus they are the best candidates for consideration of this course. In most cases, the information about hormone receptors and Her2/neu is obtained from the needle biopsy specimen, so decision making for doing chemotherapy first can be made based on the biopsy results before any surgery is performed.

NEED TO KNOW

In some patients, tumors can have an excellent response to chemotherapy, shrinking dramatically and even melting away entirely. When a tumor seemingly disappears after chemotherapy, it *does not* mean that you won't need surgery or further treatment. It does mean that surgery will be easier, and perhaps less extensive.

THE TAKEAWAY

- Chemotherapy is an important part of treatment for many women. And while all chemo regimens have side effects, these are only potential, not certain, and can range from mild to more severe.
- Endocrine or hormonal therapy is an important part of treatment for most women with hormone-receptor-positive cancer.
- A medical oncologist who specializes in breast cancer is the best person to help you make these critical decisions regarding treatment.

CHAPTER 10

Radiation

if all the cancer was removed with surgery,

why do we need it?

Picture your kitchen dishwasher. Why do you put a dish in the dishwasher even after you've rinsed it under the faucet? Well, because the dishwasher washes the plates at higher temperatures, sterilizing them and removing any spots you might have missed while rinsing. The same is true for radiation after surgery. Surgery is the main rinse—the plate under the faucet—that removes the vast majority of the cancer. The radiation—the plate in the dishwasher—then blasts away any scattered cells that may remain.

Lumpectomy and radiation usually go hand in hand, as a package deal, with surgery first and radiation to follow. In big studies involving large numbers of women, lumpectomy with radiation was found to have equivalent survival rates to mastectomy, and the risk of cancer coming back has been found to be lower than 5 percent. *Without* radiation, however, the risk of recurrence is 30 to 40 percent. In other words, if you skip radiation after lumpectomy, the chance of cancer recurrence in the same breast for most women is probably unacceptably high.

Radiation: what to expect

Radiation is a relatively short treatment: typically a few minutes of radiation five days a week for around six weeks. The treatment itself involves short bursts of radiation aimed at the breast and sometimes the armpit in order to kill any residual cancer cells in that area. During treatment, you will be lying on a firm treatment table in a very specific, still position while radiation beams are aimed at the breast. You will not feel or see anything during treatment, but you may hear the whirring of the machine, which can be loud. Each radiation treatment lasts approximately five minutes (once you are checked in and positioned), and then you can get up, leave, and proceed with your day.

Radiation treatment usually begins a minimum of three weeks after surgery so that you have time for the surgical wounds to heal. For patients who will be receiving chemotherapy after surgery, radiation is put off until after *both* surgery and chemotherapy are done. In other words, treatments for breast cancer are given sequentially, one after the other, not simultaneously. For patients who are getting surgery, chemotherapy, and radiation, it can feel like a very long haul, with treatment lasting close to a year. But you will have a few weeks' break between each type of treatment, allowing the body to recover.

Of all the treatments, radiation is perhaps the most logistically taxing, as you have to go to the hospital or clinic every day, but it is also relatively easy to endure, with minimal short-term side effects. When and if you need radiation, you will first meet with a radiation oncologist, preferably one who specializes in treatment for breast cancer. A radiation oncologist should not be confused with a radiologist (breast imaging specialist), which is a completely different kind of doctor. With radiation, there is a planning phase that usually takes a few hours, called simulation, where the radiation oncologist takes pictures of the breast and chest wall, usually with a CT scanner. These pictures enable the radiation oncologist to target the radiation beams to the breast tissue, with a focus around the area of the tumor bed, while avoiding most of the underlying chest wall, lungs, and heart.

The logistics: dealing with hospital visits

Many women have radiation at the same center or hospital where they have their surgery and chemotherapy, keeping it all under the same roof. But for some, it's more practical to receive treatment closer to home. Where I practice in New York City, many women come from outside of the city to have their surgery, but then when it comes time to have their radiation, they choose someplace nearby home so that it is more convenient and less disruptive to everyday life and their normal routine. Many of my patients find a good place to get radiation where they can stop by on their way to work. One patient of mine joked that she was tempted to just keep the car running (drive-through radiation!), and came up with the brilliant idea of combining radiation service with an ATM and food to go. Your surgeon should be able to direct you to good, solid radiation facilities in your area.

Some patients find ways to create a silver lining out of all the traveling back and forth. For example, one of my patients lived outside of New York City but decided she wanted to follow through with her treatment at our center in Manhattan. She took the train into Grand Central Terminal every day and power-walked the fifty blocks (about two and a half miles) to her radiation, and by the end of treatment she had lost ten pounds and made major progress toward her goal of a healthier lifestyle. Absolutely, it can be challenging to get to radiation every day for the many women who already have too much on their plates: jobs, kids, and other obligations can make it seem hard to fit even one more daily activity on the agenda. But the short-term commitment will lead to the best outcomes from breast cancer and the highest likelihood of never hearing from it again.

The side effects

Unlike chemotherapy, where side effects can be more severe and variable, for most people radiation treatment is fairly easy to tolerate, with the main inconvenience being that you have to get to the hospital or clinic every day. Although hair loss and nausea are *not* side effects of radiation the way they are with many chemotherapy treatments, there are some short-term side effects involved. These include

- Fatigue, especially toward the end of the six weeks and particularly in older women. Rest definitely helps. Soon after treatment ends, the fatigue abates.
- Short-term tanning or burning of the skin of the breast, which can give it a thickened, leathery appearance and feel. Sometimes the skin may peel, as if you have sunburn. The breast skin may be sensitive during treatment, and should not be exposed to the sun during and in the weeks after treatment. Many radiation oncologists prescribe or recommend topical creams that help prevent peeling and are soothing to the skin. These skin changes usually resolve over time.
- Longer-term skin damage affecting breast reconstruction. In the unlikely event that you need a mastectomy and reconstructive surgery sometime in the future—because of a cancer recurrence—you should be aware that skin damage caused by radiation could make reconstruction of the breast more complicated. Even though in most cases the skin appears to fully recover and may look exactly the same as before radiation, on a microscopic level radiation-related changes make the skin less elastic, which makes it more difficult for the skin to accommodate a tissue expander or implant (see chapter 7 on reconstruction with implants). Thankfully, recurrence rates after lumpectomy and radiation are low, and so most women do not have to face this potential scenario, but it's still important to know up front.
- Increased risk of lymphedema (see chapter 5). For women who have had an axillary dissection (all their lymph nodes removed), there is a risk of lymphedema of approximately 20 to 30 percent. For women who have had an axillary dissection and then require further radiation to the armpit area as well as the breast due to having more advanced disease, the risk of lymphedema is compounded and can be as high as 40 to 50 percent. There should not typically be a higher risk of lymphedema for those who have had only a few lymph nodes removed, as is the case with sentinel lymph node biopsy.

There are also other, more serious implications for people receiving radiation treatment. Keep in mind that these are very rarely seen with modern radiation technology, where the treatment is delivered in a more targeted and focused way than it was in decades past. In fact, the likelihood of developing a serious side effect is extremely low—affecting less than 1 percent of patients—and so in the big picture, the benefits of radiation by far outweigh the risks for the vast majority of patients who undergo it. However, it's always good to know about any serious risks up front, so for radiation, these include

- Heart and lung damage. There is an extremely low risk that when radiation beams are aimed at the breast and therefore the chest wall, there can be damage to the underlying lung or, if the cancer is in the left breast, to the heart. Both risks are less than 1 percent.
- Secondary cancer. Most people know that while radiation cures cancer, it can also cause some cancers, so there can be a small risk of developing a secondary cancer, such as skin cancer or a chest wall tumor, as a result of the radiation treatment. Again, the risk is extremely low, less than 1 percent, and so we usually do not do any special follow-up tests, other than just physical examination, to monitor for these very rare occurrences.

Radiation: the variables

A well-trained radiation oncologist in a leading center that offers cutting-edge treatments should be able to determine the appropriate regimen for each individual patient, offering you alternatives when appropriate based on the details of your case. Here are some of the considerations.

When radiation *isn't* given with lumpectomy

For some women, lumpectomy alone, without radiation, is a reasonable option. For example, a major study has shown that women over the age of seventy with smaller tumors, clear margins, negative nodes, and estrogen-receptor-positive disease have a low risk of cancer recurring in the breast, even without radiation (less than 10 percent, and there was no difference in survival rates). In addition, some women with really small, low-grade DCIS and widely clear margins may be able to forgo radiation. But most cases do not meet these conditions, and radiation is almost always recommended after lumpectomy.

There are also reasons why some women *can't* have radiation. The main reasons are

1. A full cycle of radiation treatment can be given only once to any given area. So if a woman has a lumpectomy and radiation, and is in the small, unlucky percentage of patients where the cancer comes back in the same breast, radiation can't be given again. If lumpectomy and radiation didn't work long-term the first time, there is no reason to suspect that lumpectomy alone would work the second, and this is why mastectomy is the standard treatment for patients who have recurrence within the breast.
2. Women who have had what's called mantle radiation to the chest wall for Hodgkin's disease usually cannot be radiated again, and thus mastectomy is usually the best choice for surgical treatment in this situation.
3. Women who are morbidly obese (typically greater than 300 to 350 pounds) may not be able to receive radiation, depending on their size and the weight capacity of the radiation table.
4. There are also rural areas of this country where radiation treatment is not readily available at a distance that would be feasible to travel every day for six weeks. As a result, some women choose to undergo mastectomy just to avoid the logistical challenge of the six weeks of treatment.

When shorter courses of treatment are given

While the standard radiation treatment regimen in this country is six weeks, there are some newer regimens where the patient can receive a higher percentage of the overall dose in each treatment, thereby reducing the radiation course to three weeks or even shorter. Recent data from a Canadian study showed that many women can be eligible to receive the three-week course of treatment with equivalently low risk of cancer recurrence, and this regimen is now being offered more widely across the United States as well. Some treatment methods can even deliver the entire radiation treatment intra-operatively at the time of your lumpectomy surgery, extending your surgery time by around two hours. While many of these newer types of treatments hold promise and are even offered as standard options in some centers, they are not yet standard for *all* patients. Long-term data showing their effectiveness is not yet available, and so these alternative treatment options need to be evaluated on a case-by-case basis.

There are some circumstances where this type of shorter treatment may be considered advantageous. For women who live in rural areas and have to travel great distances back and forth to the hospital site, reducing treatment from six weeks to three, or giving it all at once intra-operatively, may actually make radiation feasible when it otherwise would not be. Women who may not be able to afford time off work or the child care necessary to receive daily treatment may also truly benefit from a reduced schedule. Older women who are less mobile and who may struggle with traveling to the hospital site for treatment on a daily basis may be candidates as well. However, in general, six weeks remains the recommendation for the majority of patients.

When radiation is needed after mastectomy

While radiation is almost always given after lumpectomy, it is not commonly given after mastectomy. After a mastectomy, radiation is recommended only where there may be a risk that microscopic disease has been left behind even after the whole breast and/or lymph nodes have been completely removed. These situations include more advanced cases, when the tumor is very large, where there was invasion of the cancer into the underlying muscle or overlying skin, or if the starting diagnosis was inflammatory breast cancer. It's also important to know that radiation is also usually recommended if a large amount of cancer has spread to the lymph nodes, typically four or more, regardless of whether one has had a lumpectomy or a mastectomy. So while there is a low likelihood of needing radiation after a mastectomy, your surgeon or the oncologist who will be treating you will know if you need this. Given that radiation treatment after mastectomy would come last, after surgery and chemotherapy, these first two specialists will send you to see a radiation oncologist if need be.

THE TAKEAWAY

- Radiation reduces the rate of breast cancer coming back in the breast, and goes hand in hand with lumpectomy.
- Radiation treatment is safe, with minor side effects, and a few very rare major ones.
- *Not* receiving radiation when it is recommended highly increases the risk of recurrence.

CHAPTER 11

Sign Me Up

when participating in research or a clinical trial today
might give you the best treatment of tomorrow

When my patient Diana was diagnosed with breast cancer, she was fifty-nine and her cancer was fairly advanced. The good news was that her cancer was also curable and treatable, and so we went ahead with her surgery. After surgery, Diana saw an oncologist who told her she would need chemotherapy and that while she would receive the standard treatment, she could also participate in a clinical trial in which she would possibly receive a new drug. She called my office for advice: should she participate in the trial? She was unsure about subjecting herself to a treatment that was experimental and part of a research study.

I explained to Diana that *every* standard treatment for breast cancer was once an experiment and part of a research study in the past. The standard chemotherapy regimen that she was about to receive was once considered "experimental" until a trial showed it worked better than the previously existing treatments. In fact, research and clinical trials are the *only* way for scientists to figure out if a new treatment actually works—without them, we would never discover the best treatments of tomorrow, increase cure rates, and continue the trajectory of improved survival and more reasons for optimism.

I'm extremely supportive of clinical trials when they are appropriate for a particular patient. In this case, I encouraged Diana to participate in the trial, as the preliminary studies had been quite promising. I explained that she would get the chemotherapy treatment that had already been recommended, and then she would have a fifty-fifty chance of receiving an additional drug that could be of further benefit. The trial in question was to be a blind trial (more on what this means below), so she would not know if she was receiving the new medication until after the trial was over. The drug did have some side effects, as all medications do, but these were quite mild in most cases. And if she was picked to receive the drug, it could help reduce her risk of breast cancer recurrence, which would possibly directly benefit Diana, as well as many women in the future. Ultimately, Diana decided to participate in the trial. Although that drug has yet to become part of standard treatment, early results look extremely promising, and Diana tells me that she feels proud she was able to give back to the cancer community in this way.

Advantages and disadvantages of participating in a trial

By and large, I do recommend that my patients participate in trials if possible. Without patient participation, there would be no further advancement or improvement in treating cancer, and the generations of the future would be no better off than we are today.

Of course every volunteer who signs up for a clinical trial has to weigh the risks against the benefits. Here are some factors to keep in mind.

On the upside:

- It's an opportunity to be an active participant in your health care.
- You may gain access to cutting-edge research treatments before they're available as standard treatment.
- Some patients on clinical trials actually get better care, as they may be monitored more closely than patients on standard treatments.
- You get the feel-good factor of knowing you are benefiting women in the future by contributing to medical research.

On the downside:

- There may be added side effects—and you need to discuss these carefully with your doctor.
- The treatment simply may not work.
- The treatment may take up more of your time than a standard treatment, with additional tests and visits to the doctor.
- You might not actually get the medication if you're in the group that gets a placebo; you won't know until the trial is over.

MYTH: "When you offer to be a guinea pig, you're going to be treated like a guinea pig."

When you offer to participate in a trial or research, this does not mean you are being experimented on like a lab animal. In most cases, only the top institutions and top doctors offer trials to their patients, since these are the places where the newer, better treatments start out. There are very stringent rules governing medical trials that ensure fairness, safety, and adequacy of treatment. Most trials usually offer a standard treatment along with a newer treatment option that may be even better and not yet available outside of a trial. In other words, you're less likely to be treated like a guinea pig and more likely to be treated like a VIP.

Participating in a trial: questions to ask before participating

- How long will the trial last?
- How often will I need to come to the hospital?
- What are the side effects?
- What are the possible benefits to me—and to women in the future?
- What is the long-term goal of the trial?
- How are you going to monitor me and my safety during the trial? Will there be extra blood tests? Scans? If so, how frequently?
- How will my medical information be used and will it remain private?
- Who is paying for the trial?

- Are you—my doctor—receiving any financial incentive to introduce patients to this trial? (See the note on financial compensation below.)
- What are the endpoints of the trial?
- Are there any circumstances in which I might be taken off the trial along the way?

Red flags: when to walk away

If you agree to participate in a clinical trial, you should make sure that your questions are being answered from the outset, and that there are personnel available whom you can check in with along the way if issues arise. If you feel that you're not getting the information you need, then you are fully within your rights to decline to participate and/or discontinue participation. Also, if personal circumstances prevent you from feeling comfortable participating in a trial, you shouldn't feel coerced or that the quality of your care will suffer if you do walk away. (For more on clinical trials and listings of trials, see the list of online resources at the back of the book.)

Participating in a trial: What to expect

1. **Informed consent.** When you are considering participation in a clinical trial, the process usually involves a lengthy explanation from your doctor or the principal investigator (leader of the trial) describing the rationale for the trial and why it might make sense for you to participate. You may need to agree to additional tests or to give further information to determine if you meet the eligibility criteria for the trial. If you do meet the criteria, you would then be asked to sign a paper saying that you give informed consent—essentially, that the risks and benefits of the trial have been discussed with you and that you are freely agreeing to participate. This is standard procedure; you don't need a lawyer to vet this document!
2. **The randomization process.** In general, different trials involve different interventions. For example, some trials compare a standard treatment to a placebo (a sugar pill or inactive treatment).

These trials, where there is potentially no actual treatment given, are never done in patients who actually need treatment. Some trials compare a standard treatment with or without one added drug or treatment to determine its added benefit. As scientists, we can't find out if a new medication is more effective by simply giving the drug to patients. We have to scientifically compare two similar groups of patients receiving different treatments in order to see who has better outcomes over the long term. As such, many research studies involve a randomization process, whereby each individual who agrees to participate is randomly assigned—usually by a computer program—to one arm or the other of the trial. This increases the likelihood that patient characteristics such as age, severity of disease, and overall health will not be biased toward one arm of the trial, which could then affect the objectivity of the results. So the randomization process is done to create a level playing field when evaluating two different types of treatment, and to make sure that results from the trial accurately reflect, as much as possible, the true effects of the treatments given.

3. **The trial itself.** During the trial, you and your doctor may or may not know whether or not you are receiving the additional treatment, depending on whether or not the trial is blinded. In a blind trial, the doctor, patient, or both do not know which arm of the trial they are on, and whether or not they are receiving the experimental treatment; this ensures that benefits and side effects that the doctors and patients report are not biased or related to placebo effect (the phenomenon of feeling better even when your medication or pill is a sugar pill). For example, one large, important trial that was done in the 1990s and reported results in 1999 investigated whether or not tamoxifen, a medication that is frequently given to patients to treat their breast cancer, could also have a preventive effect for women who are at increased risk for developing the disease. The trial involved approximately thirteen thousand women at increased risk for breast cancer who were randomized into two groups, evenly matched for their risk, age, and other factors. During the trial half received tamoxifen and the other half received a placebo. At the end of the study pe-

riod, the tamoxifen group developed almost 50 percent fewer new breast cancers than those assigned to placebo. The dramatic results of this study led to immediate early cessation of the trial so that results could be reported and women on the placebo could switch over to tamoxifen, potentially also reducing their future risk. But here's why it was so important that the trial included a placebo group. Tamoxifen does have side effects, many of which are subjective in nature, including (so we thought) weight gain. But the placebo group, who did not know whether they were on tamoxifen or not, actually gained more weight overall than the tamoxifen group. These findings objectively demonstrated that in general, tamoxifen is *not* associated with substantial weight gain. Had the trial not included a placebo and/or not been blinded, there would have been no way of knowing whether or not the weight gain was clearly a result of taking tamoxifen or not.*

4. **Concluding the trial.** Usually trials play out over the course of months to years; they are expensive to run, and they require huge amounts of data processing to ascertain results. Often, if it becomes clear that the treatment is beneficial, as was the case with the tamoxifen trial described above, the trial will end ahead of time so that everyone can benefit from the new finding as soon as possible. Equally, if the trial clearly shows there has been no benefit to patients, or if the side effects are more serious or detrimental than expected, the trial may be stopped early. Otherwise a trial typically proceeds to its conclusion with extensive continued monitoring for side effects, overall health, and disease recurrence. Some patients do not complete a trial due to disproportionate side effects, or based on a clear-cut lack of benefit. The decision to come off a trial is one you would make with your doctor along the way. If for some reason you can't complete a trial, this should not be viewed as a failure in any way; indeed,

* Fisher B, Costantino JP, Wickerham DL, et al. Tamoxifen for prevention of breast cancer: report of the National Surgical Adjuvant Breast and Bowel Project P-1 Study. *Journal of the National Cancer Institute,* 1998.

your experience with the trial, one way or the other, will help the trial scientists learn more about breast cancer.

A note on financial compensation

There are usually no significant financial benefits to patients for research participation, although sometimes patients are offered some modest compensation for their time or travel expenses incurred as a result of participation. What's more, there also really should not be any significant compensation or financial incentive for the doctor to put you on a clinical trial, as this would be considered a conflict of interest. You want your doctor to be looking out for you and making the best recommendations for your care without any consideration for how it might benefit him or her in other ways. And you should feel comfortable confirming with your doctor that he or she has no potential financial benefit that might encourage him or her to push you toward participation. For example, owning stock in the company that sells the drug in the trial, or consulting for a company that pays consulting fees to doctors are two ways that doctors could financially benefit from encouraging trial participation.

THE TAKEAWAY

- Clinical trials today are the key to better treatment options tomorrow.
- Participating in research is not in any way tantamount to becoming a guinea pig. If you are offered the chance to participate, give it careful consideration and move forward knowing that you will be monitored closely.
- Always get a detailed description of the potential risks and benefits, and make sure you understand them.

CHAPTER 12

Recovery After Treatment

ongoing care

For many patients, the period after breast cancer treatment ends is a surprisingly challenging one. You might think that after completing what could be months of treatment, every patient would simply pop open a bottle of champagne and move on. For most women, however, the range of emotions can be much more complex. Yes, there's the initial sense of triumph, but after the high, there's often a period of feeling very low. You may look and feel very different. You may have undergone a dramatic physical change such as a mastectomy or hair loss. And despite the misconception that women lose weight from cancer and chemotherapy, it's actually quite common for some women to gain weight as a side effect of some of the treatments (and because you may have less energy and therefore engage in less activity during the treatment period). Even if your particular treatment plan did not result in significant physical changes visible from the outside, your sense of yourself as invulnerable and always healthy will certainly have changed in some way, forever.

Now that you're no longer seeing your doctors on such a regular basis, you may experience feelings of despair and confusion. One patient explained it to me this way: "Ever since my treatment finished, I don't feel that I'm being protected from the cancer anymore." I've also seen patients who struggle with maintaining patience during the recovery period. I had one patient who runs marathons. During and after her chemotherapy, however, she was too tired and too drained to run for a period of weeks. She found it very demoralizing to slow down, and we spent a lot of time during her recovery period talking about patience and about taking some time for the healing to happen. Another patient was a reporter who worked for a worldwide news agency and traveled regularly to report from all parts of the planet, wherever the latest conflict took her. After she finished surgery and was about to start chemotherapy, I warned her that she might want to cut herself some slack and sit out some of the intense traveling while undergoing treatment. There would be no shortage of bigger stories in the future, I suggested. She sort of smirked at my comment, as if to say, "We'll just see about that." About two months later, around the time she was finishing her fourth cycle of chemotherapy, I was home with my family eating dinner and the news was on. I recognized the voice coming from the screen, and looked up to see my patient reporting from Moscow—in her wig and a baseball cap. What did I know about patience and recovery? When it came to her case, apparently not much.

The point is that there is no fixed timetable or script to follow when it comes to the pace of your personal recovery, and there is certainly no need to rush. Whatever type or types of treatment you have, it can help to keep in mind that the physical recovery from any type of breast surgery and treatment is much like recovery from an injury. If you sprain your ankle, you don't go out the next day and run four miles. Usually you rest it for a period of time, and then, when you are ready, you start back slowly, listen to your body, and build up strength over time. That's how it works with cancer recovery—it's slow to begin with, but over time you begin to feel better and stronger. Most women who were healthy and active in the first place can return to their baseline level of function. It just takes time. Here is a summary of some of the physical, mental, and emotional aspects of recovery that patients tell me about every day.

Physical recuperation—surgery, chemotherapy, radiation

Lumpectomy. Lumpectomy surgery, with or without sentinel node biopsy, requires some recuperation, but physical recovery is usually fairly rapid. Because it is a short procedure, there is almost never an overnight stay in the hospital, which means you will be up and around almost immediately after surgery. While you may be a bit sore, you will be able to do most of your usual activities on your own, including eating, going to the bathroom, and getting dressed without any assistance. Many of my lumpectomy patients who have office jobs return to work within a couple of days. Driving might be associated with a bit of discomfort because of the arm movement involved in turning the steering wheel, especially if you have had lymph nodes removed under your arm, but this soreness should not last for long. Work or activities that involve a higher level of physical activity, such as lifting heavy things, moving things, heavy cleaning, or exercise, may require a bit more of a recovery period, two to three weeks, before you can fully return to those functions.

If you have a lumpectomy, you can expect a complete return to your baseline function, and there is usually no change in sensation in the breast or nipple. Occasionally patients complain of a pulling or tightening sensation within the breast even years later, perhaps from scar tissue, but these sensations, which can come and go, usually do not affect overall quality of life or function in any major way.

Mastectomy. Mastectomy or bilateral mastectomy involves a longer physical recovery period than lumpectomy, usually four to six weeks. The length and intensity of the recovery period also depends on the type of reconstruction, if any, you have chosen to have. (For more details on the different types of reconstruction, refer to chapter 7.) Mastectomy, with or without implant surgery, requires a hospital stay of one to two nights. While mastectomy is definitely a major surgical operation, we only remove skin and soft tissue and don't cut through muscle, as with abdominal surgery or surgery within the chest cavity. As a result, most women can be up and around and using their core abdominal muscles to sit up, even the day of surgery. Full activity in four to six weeks is the norm.

Mastectomy with a flap reconstruction usually requires a three- to five-night stay in the hospital, since taking tissue from another part of the body involves recovery of the donor site as well. For women who have a mastectomy and abdominal flap reconstruction, recovery would be similar to that of having a tummy tuck at the same time as breast surgery, which means greater initial immobility and a longer total recovery period (perhaps six weeks or longer).

For mastectomy with either type of reconstruction, it can take a while to adjust to new sensations, or lack thereof, such as numbness along the chest wall and where the nipple used to be.

A WORD TO THE WISE

Mastectomy surgery may also lead many women to reassess their wardrobes. If you don't have reconstruction, you will most likely wear a prosthesis made of foam or gel in your bra to fill out the cup. With the prosthesis and post-mastectomy bra, most clothing, including many one-piece bathing suits, can be worn in exactly the same way without anyone noticing any outward change at all, but wearing certain kinds of clothing items can be a challenge. For example, strapless dresses are tough without a breast to hold one side up: one patient of mine had to rethink her mother-of-the-bride dress when she had a mastectomy about one month before her daughter's wedding. If you do have reconstruction, then you may find that your breasts are much "perkier" than before. The new shape and size of your breasts can definitely influence what you choose to wear: either more or less revealing, including in the bathing suit and lingerie departments.

For many women who are recovering from breast cancer surgery, especially mastectomy, feeling self-conscious is natural, especially when it comes to intimate relationships and being naked. There is no question: your new breast (or breasts) will look and feel different. It's also important to remember that reconstruction is a process, so your appearance may be something of a work in progress for the first few months after surgery. When it comes to intimate relationships, communication of course is key: you and your partner should be able to speak about the changes that will affect both of you before, during, and after the process. There is no question that such surgery comes with adjustments, and getting used to the new appearance and sensations (or lack of sensation) can take time for you *and* for your partner. The good news is that many of my patients have told me that they have a newfound closeness with their partner after going through the trauma of a cancer diagnosis and coming out the other end together.

Axillary Dissection

Recovery from the larger axillary dissection surgery involves maintaining some degree of vigilance against the development of lymphedema (arm swelling related to the removal of a large number of lymph nodes under the arm; see chapter 5 for more details). Approximately 20 to 30 percent of women who have all their lymph nodes removed will develop lymphedema. This risk increases to 40 to 50 percent when the lymph nodes are removed *and* subsequent radiation directed to the armpit is also needed. Lymphedema can develop at any time, with or without known triggers. Events that can increase the risk of lymphedema include anything that puts the hand or arm on the affected side at risk for infection, any arm activity that is exhaustive and repetitive, and any type of garment or activity that restricts blood and lymphatic flow to the forearm or hand. I usually advise my patients who have their lymph nodes removed to be aware, but not obsessive, about the risk of lymphedema. If signs do develop, then early intervention with massage and arm elevation can help alleviate symptoms. For some women, particularly obese and diabetic women, lymphedema is a lifetime struggle, but it's important to know that while this condition can be uncomfortable, unsightly, and unwieldy, it is not life-threatening for the vast majority of women. In very rare circumstances, women with chronic lymphedema can develop a specific type of cancer of the lymph system in the arm, called lymphangiosarcoma. Again, this is extremely rare and not something to worry about for most women. Whichever doctor continues to monitor you over the long term will check you for signs of lymphedema and its potential complications.

Recovery from chemotherapy and hormonal therapy

During recovery after chemotherapy, your hair will start to grow back, which for many women is the first triumphant sign that a significant part of treatment is over. Most women do recover from chemotherapy completely, but there are a range of different side effects that can stay with you, including neuropathy (numbness or pain, especially in the fingertips, feet, and toes), menopausal-type side effects (including hot flashes and long-term effects on fertility), and the dreaded "chemo-brain" (for more on all of these, refer to chapter 9). Some chemotherapy agents are even associated with a small increased risk of secondary cancers such as leukemia. It's important to know that side effects are potential, not certain or even likely.

For hormonal therapy, the treatment is long-term, and changes after cessation of medication are minimal. Recovery from chemotherapy is gradual, with an increasing feeling of returning to normal over the ensuing weeks after treatment ends. It's also important to keep in mind as you recover that some women who develop unwanted side effects experience feelings of regret over taking treatment. It's natural to wonder if perhaps you should have opted not to take a certain treatment so that you wouldn't have to live with the side effects. When it comes to the years of hormonal treatment, some women even consider discontinuing treatment to reduce the side effects they experience. But having regrets and second-guessing yourself is never very productive. And it's critical to keep in mind the key fact that these treatments were considered necessary to increase your chances of survival from breast cancer. So instead of regret, you can derive some peace of mind from knowing that you have done everything you can to give yourself the best possible outcome for the long term.

Recovery from radiation

For the most part, radiation affects your skin and your energy levels, and so after treatment ends, you will begin to see resolution of the skin changes, and increased energy. When radiation concludes, you can also return to your usual routine without the drudgery of travel to your daily radiation appointment, which after six weeks can be extremely liberating. Interestingly, because radiation is often the last type of treatment given, finishing radiation can often signify the true completion of active treatment, and become associated with a wave of feelings totally disproportionate to what you might expect.

Emotional recuperation: what to expect

Although cancer is a physical disease, there is no doubt that fighting breast cancer takes patients on an intensely emotional journey. From the initial shock of diagnosis to the stress of undergoing treatment to the joy of the cancer being eradicated, most patients find themselves experiencing the full gamut of emotions. This psychological journey continues after active treatment is over too. Part of the struggle for patients has to do with figuring out the "new normal." Yes, the goal is for any cancer patient to get back to normal life, but more often this means reestablishing your sense of what normal means to you *now*. Your new normal may mean living with some fear of cancer recurrence. Your new normal may mean being much more aware of your health than you ever were before. The new normal may also mean you have a fresh outlook on life and a deeper appreciation of everything you may have previously taken for granted. For many patients, this leads to a reevaluation of their priorities, resulting in positive and dramatic changes. Jobs, relationships, hobbies, charity work, religious affiliation or spirituality—for most of my patients, their outlook on life becomes subject to at least some reassessment and change. My advice is to listen to your feelings; don't try to override them or "get over" cancer right away. Over time, the experience of cancer will fade into the background and you will begin to find your way forward again. And if you find yourself still struggling to adapt a year or more down the line, you may want to consider seeking professional emotional support, either from a group of other survivors or from a trained counselor.

Your follow-up regimen

After the active treatment phase is over, every doctor has his or her own preferred follow-up regimen. Most see patients every three to four months to start, transitioning to twice a year and ultimately once a year. The problem arises when you have multiple doctors involved in your care and each doctor wants to see you two or three times a year— you can quickly end up with doctor appointment overload! It's hard to return to normal life if you are dragging yourself to the surgeon, the medical oncologist, or the radiation oncologist every month.

If it's possible, you can ask your doctors to coordinate your visits. Perhaps you will see your surgeon once a year, every January, and then see your medical oncologist once a year, every July. This way, you are receiving continuous care from all your doctors while appropriately spacing out the visits. On the other hand, you don't want to feel abandoned by your doctors, and most breast cancer surgeons and oncologists *do* see their patients regularly in follow-up for at least a few years after treatment.

Breast cancer survivorship programs

Many centers and hospitals that treat breast cancer patients will have a "survivorship" program that you can join after a varying number of years, usually starting a minimum of two years post-treatment. Survivorship programs are a great way to continue with cancer care follow-up while still moving forward with a focus on overall health. A good survivorship program will help you get back up to date on other basic health checks such as Pap smears and colonoscopies (many cancer patients fall behind on other basic and routine exams during cancer treatment). In addition, if there are any long-term side effects related to your cancer treatment, survivorship caregivers—who are often MDs but can also be physician assistants or nurse practitioners working under the supervision of the doctor—are trained to watch and screen for these. Many survivorship programs also are able to refer you to support groups, psychologists, and psychiatrists if you feel you might want this added support.

Recommendations for follow-up tests

Once you've completed treatment for cancer, it's normal to be concerned that the cancer will come back. *Every* woman who comes to my office post-treatment wants to discuss testing going forward: "Shouldn't I get more frequent scans and tests of the body to find out if the cancer has come back so it can be detected early?" The answer is that unless you underwent a bilateral mastectomy, where both breasts have been removed, then yes, we need to continue with screening. This will include appropriate breast imaging tests and physical examinations— usually on a yearly basis, but sometimes twice a year for the first two years after treatment.

Oftentimes it's your surgeon who will make sure appropriate imaging studies of the breasts and physical examinations are being performed going forward. He or she knows your case the best and can determine if any changes on your physical exam are cause for concern. Some patients will also need to add ultrasounds or MRIs to their screening regimen (see chapter 1 for more information about screening and decision making about additional studies). It's important to remember that if your cancer was missed by a mammogram the first time, this does not necessarily mean your mammogram would miss a cancer the *second* time, so you may not necessarily need every test available to screen for recurrence. Furthermore, unless you had a bilateral mastectomy, you do still need a yearly mammogram, whether your cancer was or was not detected by mammogram the first time, as mammography is still the best way to detect recurrence the earliest in most women.

A WORD TO THE WISE

Scanning for recurrence: when more testing isn't better
When it comes to early detection of local recurrence (in the breast), some patients do need a more frequent screening schedule in the ensuing year or two following surgery. And adding tests such as ultrasound or MRI to mammograms may be appropriate for some, but not all, and should be discussed with your doctor. The ultimate goal, however, is to return you to a schedule of yearly mammography. Why is this? For most of my patients, going back to annual mammograms feels counterintuitive: "I've had breast cancer, so I should be screening as much as possible to make sure we catch the cancer early if it comes back!" In general, it's impor-

tant to know that more testing is *not* always better and does come with a potential price: the more tests you have, the greater the risk of the tests showing false positive findings.

The same is true for scans of the body looking for cancer recurrence. Imagine you have a CT scan of the body after having breast cancer and the results show some tiny dot on the lung. Unless you had regular CT scans from years prior to your diagnosis, we have no way of knowing if this dot was there before the breast cancer or if it's a new cancer that's growing within the body. The dot may be a scar or something completely benign. Or not. If this dot is big enough, your doctor may recommend a biopsy, which involves either a major lung operation or a needle biopsy, both of which are associated with substantial risks. If the dot is too small to find on a biopsy, your doctor will usually recommend waiting three to six months and getting another scan to see if the dot grew. Neither option is particularly attractive: either you need a major interventional procedure to find out if the dot on your lung means your cancer has spread, or you are going to spend the next few months of your life stressed and anxious while you wait for the next test. And most important, finding a spot on the lung that *is* breast cancer spread in no way represents early detection or increases the likelihood of successful treatment for metastatic breast cancer.

So before you go to your doctor demanding tests and scans to quell your anxiety that your cancer has come back, understand that more tests are usually not a great antidote for your fears of recurrence, and can end up doing more harm than good.

Tumor markers: a cautionary tale

My patient Kate was doing really well post-treatment. Her breast cancer diagnosis was three years in the past and she was back to her old active life. Kate was seeing me every six months and her oncologist every six months for routine exams and getting mammograms once a year. Then she went for a routine visit with her primary care doctor, who told Kate that in addition to her existing screening regimen with me and her oncologist, she should really get her tumor markers checked.

Tumor markers are a type of blood test that can be valuable tools for screening *some* types of cancer survivors (those who have had prostate cancer, for example) to determine whether the cancer has come back. For breast cancer survivors, however, tumor markers are not a very accurate test, since there are many factors that can affect marker levels that have nothing to do with cancer (smoking, infection, and so forth). While in select patients tumor markers can be useful to track response to treatment and monitor those at high risk for recurrence, we also know that for most women they are *not* useful or helpful. In fact, tumor markers can be completely normal in women with breast cancer and completely abnormal in women with no breast cancer! For this reason, these tumor markers are *not* recommended as part of routine follow-up for *most* women who have had breast cancer.

Kate's primary care physician felt otherwise, though, and so he explained to her that it must have been an oversight that we hadn't ordered the test. He immediately drew blood on Kate and sent it out to be tested for tumor markers. The normal range for tumor markers is 31 or under. Kate's result came back at 33. And that's when Kate called me, frantic. Though she had been feeling perfectly well and happy, she was now understandably scared out of her mind.

Kate came in to see us and we scanned her from head to toe. When the scans revealed nothing specific or concerning, we explained to her that this was reassuring but that we would have to recheck the blood test again in a month or two, and if the results continued to trend upward, we might need to repeat the scans, since in some cases elevated tumor markers can precede the manifestation of metastatic disease.

Needless to say, the next month was not a happy time for Kate. She found it impossible to focus on anything other than the possibility that the cancer had come back. She was having headaches now. Were these a result of the extreme stress she was experiencing, or were they, heaven forbid, related to brain metastases? It was awful watching someone go through this, especially when she had been doing so well beforehand.

When we repeated the blood test a month later and the results came back at 22, well within the normal range, Kate popped open a bottle of champagne, and she sent me one too. I opened my bottle that night at home and drank a toast to her health. Sadly, my patient had to learn the hard way that every test, even something as seemingly innocuous as a blood test, has the potential to open up a can of worms without any real benefit in the long term. Why were her results elevated a month before? We will never know. But one thing was for sure: Kate and I agreed that as long as she felt healthy, there would be no more blood tests for tumor markers. Fortunately, Kate's primary care doctor got on board with the plan as well.

A WORD TO THE WISE

As you transition from actively fighting the disease to living a healthy life, you're going to have less frequent contact with your cancer treatment team. Weaning yourself off frequent doctor visits should happen gradually and is a good thing—you don't want to be a patient forever! But this time can also leave you vulnerable to chatter and second opinions from medical professionals who are not breast cancer specialists and also non-medical sources. Bonding with other breast cancer survivors who are years out from their treatment may provide welcome reassurance during your recovery period that you too can and will be a long-term survivor. But breast cancer survivors love to compare notes, and this happens in support groups, in chat rooms online, and in person. Hearing too many stories from others who underwent a different treatment or chose a different path can leave you with feelings of regret and confusion, second-guessing the very sound choices you made in the first place. This is a good time to remind yourself that when it comes to breast cancer treatment, one size does not fit all. You made the right decisions for *you* based on your specific case, in collaboration with *your* team of specialists, and you have every reason to feel confident in the care you received and the decisions you made.

THE TAKEAWAY

- Recovery takes time, mastectomy longer than lumpectomy, and some people longer than others.
- Completing treatment means less frequent visits with the doctors. Remember: this is a good thing!
- When it comes to follow-up testing, more is not always better.

CHAPTER 13

Lifestyle Factors

what do diet, stress, alcohol, and smoking

have to do with breast cancer?

When I was a surgery resident, I went through a period of working 120 hours a week (in case you were wondering, there are only 168 hours in every week). During these months of being on call and working almost nonstop, I developed what I thought was an ingenious plan to keep myself well fortified for the long, exhausting nights at the hospital. I would buy myself a big pack of M&Ms from the cafeteria vending machine at about 9:00 p.m. and go through them one by one, rationing them over the course of the night. By 6:00 a.m. I would have finished the whole pack. In my deranged, sleep-deprived mind, I developed the amusing theory that in a packet of M&Ms you had all the major food groups: the red ones were the meat group, the green ones were the vegetables, the yellow ones were the dairy, and so on. After about a month of this highly sophisticated nutritional regimen, I got out of the shower one night, rubbed my face with a towel, and immediately saw little hairs on my towel. I looked in the mirror and was horrified to find that the middle part of my right eyebrow had completely fallen out. Almost certainly this was due to my malnourished state and the lack of vitamins in my vending machine diet!

As if the embarrassment of showing up at work in my eyebrowless state was not enough, I was going on vacation out of the country a few weeks later for some much-needed R&R, but I had to renew my pass-port before I went, so my freakish appearance would be permanently documented by my new passport picture. Luckily, I remembered my grandmother's trick of "penciling it in," which somewhat concealed the problem until my eyebrow grew back (which, incidentally, takes months). The message from this story? Poor nutrition can influence health in all kinds of ways, everything from loss of eyebrow hair to increasing one's risk for cancer.

The risk factors

For many women, a cancer diagnosis can serve as a wake-up call. After treatment ends, it's very common for patients to ask about what life-style factors they can change to reduce the risk of cancer coming back—or to reduce the risk of developing another cancer. Some risk factors for cancer, such as the genes we inherit, are out of our control, but others—diet, exercise, smoking, alcohol intake, and stress—are all factors we can control, and each of them plays an important role in our overall health.

Diet

There is no question that altering your diet can play a significant role in reducing the risk of many diseases, heart disease, hypertension, and diabetes among them. Dietary factors can also play a role in the devel-opment of certain cancers, including stomach cancer, esophageal cancer, and colon cancer. When it comes to breast cancer, however, nutrition and dietary factors have been investigated extensively for their poten-tial roles in cancer development or prevention, and so far the verdict is still out: no one single dietary factor has been specifically linked as a clear-cut contributor to the development of breast cancer. Not red meat. Not fatty foods. Not too many M&Ms.

This is good news and bad news for patients. It's good news because if you have breast cancer, you can rest assured that your diet wasn't a factor and you are not at fault (no matter how much you try to blame yourself). The bad news is that there's not much that you can do from a nutritional standpoint that will reduce the risk of your cancer coming back in the future. Certainly, a healthy diet including large amounts of fresh fruits and vegetables, whole grains, and smaller amounts of animal proteins is proven to be beneficial to overall health and can possibly lower the risk of cancer in general. However, no specific dietary element has been successfully and consistently shown to reduce the risk for breast cancer.

MYTH: "Eating soy can give you breast cancer."

This is a good example of how little we know about the connection between specific dietary elements and breast cancer. Much research has been focused on soy and soy products and whether or not they increase or decrease the risk of breast cancer. The theory goes that soy looks a lot like estrogen to the body, so therefore it might increase your hormone levels, which in turn can lead to increased breast cancer risk. Other research indicates that soy might *decrease* the risk of breast cancer because the incidence of breast cancer is lower in Asian women, who in general consume diets high in soy, especially early in life. The take-home message is that there is as much research pointing to soy being associated with a *lower* risk of breast cancer as there is linking it to a *higher* risk of breast cancer, leading most doctors to conclude that eating soy is fine in moderation, which means approximately three to four servings per week.

Obesity

While no specific dietary component has been directly related to breast cancer risk or recurrence, there is one factor related to diet that is *directly* connected to breast cancer risk, and that's obesity. Obesity actively increases your risk of breast cancer, and here's why: fat stores in the body produce estrogen, and increased estrogen exposure leads to increased risk of breast cancer. There are other biologic mechanisms that have also been implicated in the obesity–breast cancer connection as well, including insulin resistance pathways and higher levels of circulating growth factors in obese people. Not only does obesity increase the risk of breast cancer; it also increases the risk of cancer coming back, specifically for women with hormone-receptor-positive disease. Recent data has shown that normal-weight women may have up to a

5 percent survival benefit over obese women—a dramatic advantage of similar magnitude to that provided by chemotherapy in some cases.

Obesity also significantly increases the risk of complications related to many aspects of breast cancer treatment. When it comes to surgery, people who are obese are more susceptible to wound infections and blood clots, and are at greater risk for complications related to anesthesia. When it comes to the medical treatment of breast cancer, obesity can also complicate your care: when chemotherapy is needed, getting IVs started is much more difficult in patients who are obese. Furthermore, the drug tamoxifen, an important medication that many women need to reduce their risk of cancer coming back, has as a side effect an increased risk of blood clots and clots traveling to the lung, a serious and potentially life-threatening complication. This occurrence is usually quite rare, but it is much more common in women who are obese. And lastly, women who are morbidly obese may not even be able to have radiation due to weight limits for the radiation table, which may mean they cannot have a lumpectomy, even if they have a small cancer.

This doesn't mean that the minute a woman receives a cancer diagnosis she needs to be told that she has to lose weight! It's stressful enough receiving the news that you have breast cancer and dealing with the ensuing treatment without adding weight loss into the equation. Many women with weight problems use eating and food for comfort and as a coping mechanism, and so again, the period after a breast cancer diagnosis may not be the best time to start a new diet.

But *after* treatment is over, many women do want to take control of their future health by reducing their weight. If a healthy diet and regular exercise aren't helping, then it may be time to talk to your doctor about alternatives.

Exercise

Exercise is an important part of overall health and can contribute to well-being in many ways. The breast cancer patients that I meet who have always exercised regularly have improved cardiovascular health and endurance, better bone density, a healthier state of mind, and a faster recovery time after surgery and treatment.

Exercise certainly helps with weight control as well, and thus may reduce the risk of breast cancer in the first place. Also, there is some evidence that young women with breast cancer who exercise heavily may have a reduction in their risk of cancer recurring (but it is unclear whether this is a cause-and-effect phenomenon or just an association—maybe these same young women who exercise also maintain a lower body weight, which may be the more important factor). Although it's difficult to tease out the specific contribution of exercise in keeping breast cancer at bay, what we do know is that exercise is important, and given national trends toward increased obesity, decreased activity, and increased consumption of unhealthy foods, there's no argument to be made for shying away from working out on a regular basis.

If you can make healthier living—including regular exercise—a priority, it can benefit you in so many ways. That doesn't mean your new regimen needs to start while you're going through cancer treatment. It's understandably difficult to make your general health a priority when you're fully engaged in the battle against breast cancer, but the goal is for the breast cancer to fade into the background at some point so that you can actually focus on your health and body as a whole. The ideal amount of exercise, frequency, and type of exercise that maximally improves health is debatable. For you, it might be a daily walk; or it might be running marathons. The optimum type of exercise is something only you can determine, based on your personal preference and in consultation with your doctor and other health professionals. The general recommendations are for thirty minutes a day of combined cardiovascular and strength training exercise.

Smoking

Smoking is evil. It's that simple. In the interest of full disclosure, I admit that my husband is a lung cancer surgeon and so I hear about the casualties of that disease every day. If I wanted to, I could fill the rest of the pages of this book describing all of the terrible things that can happen to a smoker, and it's not only lung cancer. There's throat cancer, emphysema, asthma, bronchitis, vascular disease, and heart disease, to name just a few. But this book is not about smoking and lung cancer; it's about breast cancer. And the honest truth is that one of the only diseases that *isn't* brought on by smoking is breast cancer.

That doesn't mean that if you have a breast cancer diagnosis it's fine to keep puffing away. If you are a smoker and develop early-stage breast cancer, your survival from breast cancer is, in some respects, the least of your problems relative to your overall future health. You are much more likely to die from heart disease or some other smoking-related illness than you are from your breast cancer.

But let's get back to breast cancer specifically. What we do know is that smokers with a breast cancer diagnosis often have a much harder time during surgery and recovery. Smoking decimates the small blood vessels that are critical for one side of an incision to reconnect to the other, so wound healing can take longer, and this can lead to wound breakdown and infection, which can then delay subsequent treatment. Smoking also leads to an increased risk of complications during and after surgery that are really very serious: smokers have a higher risk of developing pneumonia and other lung infections after general anesthesia. Smokers also have a higher risk of developing blood clots in the legs, which can then travel to the lungs. This phenomenon, called a pulmonary embolism, is actually potentially life threatening.

Smoking can affect your options for reconstruction if you have a mastectomy. If you are an active smoker, you may not be eligible for reconstruction performed with a flap (taking tissue from one part of the body and moving it to fill in the empty breast space) since the flap will only be successful if the blood vessel supplying the flap is viable. No plastic surgeon wants to hook up one blood vessel that is compromised by smoking to another blood vessel compromised by smoking; it's often just too risky. Surprisingly, quitting smoking for even a few weeks before surgery can potentially improve blood flow and circulation, making you a better candidate for reconstruction, and reducing your risk of postoperative complications.

Of course, telling someone to quit smoking when they have just been diagnosed with breast cancer is unlikely to have a positive effect. For one thing, you can't reverse years of smoking damage by stopping for a few weeks. For another, in the same way some people use food to cope with stress, others use smoking as a comfort mechanism, and most would find the idea of quitting at a time of maximum stress completely intolerable. I remember one patient saying to me, "Let me get this straight: you want me to deal with breast cancer *and* quit smoking?

Next you're going to tell me I have to lose thirty pounds too! It's not going to happen. Just put me out of my misery." So the bottom line is you have to do your best and be realistic about what you can handle at any given time. But understand that quitting smoking is probably just as important to your overall health as getting correct and complete treatment for breast cancer. If you are struggling with quitting smoking on your own, you should talk to your doctor about other options like medication or therapeutic techniques such as hypnosis, which can work in some cases.

Alcohol

While there's no proven link between breast cancer and dietary factors, it has been shown that there is a connection between heavy alcohol intake and an increased risk for breast cancer *and* breast cancer recurrence. This is most likely related to alcohol's adverse effect on liver function. It's the liver that helps to metabolize and break down hormones circulating in the body, especially estrogen. Therefore, if liver function is compromised, then hormones are not broken down as effectively, leading to higher levels of circulating estrogen. And higher levels of estrogen definitely increase the risk of developing breast cancer and can fuel the growth of an already present cancer. How do we define heavy alcohol intake? Most guidelines indicate that alcohol in moderation means three to five servings (drinks of any kind) a week. More than one drink a day is the approximate level at which increased risk starts. So if you do drink regularly, you may want to cut back after your breast cancer diagnosis as a way to actively take control of your future health. If you are having a hard time achieving this, then you may want to seek some professional help.

Stress and cancer

Many of my patients instinctively blame their cancer diagnosis on stress. After patients receive a diagnosis, they will frequently tell me that they "know why this happened": the stressful events in their lives are the reason they have gotten cancer. Of course it's true that modern life is stressful, and most of us feel overwhelmed much of the time, but this doesn't mean there's any clear-cut evidence that stress is a contributing factor in cancer.

Having said that, I think most of my colleagues in the medical profession would agree that there is some kind of complex relationship between stress and the immune system—and that there is a connection between the immune system and the development of cancer. So if you feel that there are regimens that you can engage in that reduce stress as part of a healthy lifestyle—meditation, yoga, or other gentle exercise, for example—then this certainly won't do you any harm.

If you *are* concerned that stress may have been a contributing factor in your cancer diagnosis and you are blaming yourself as a result, it can help to remember the following fact: many studies have been done on groups of people—including former prisoners of war and Holocaust survivors—who have been exposed to prolonged periods of extreme stress and trauma, and *none* of these groups have been shown to have any increased likelihood of developing any type of cancer.

MYTH: "Stop feeling stressed about your cancer diagnosis! You're only going to make the cancer worse."

As discussed above, *there's no proven link* between stress and breast cancer. Yet this may not stop friends and family members from advising you to "relax! You'll only make the cancer spread." Telling a stressed-out person to relax is like telling a hungry person to stop thinking about food: it just makes it worse! The bottom line is that it's completely normal to feel stressed about a cancer diagnosis. Don't make yourself feel any worse by listening to those people who tell you that your stress is a contributing factor in your disease or its spread. It's simply not the truth.

MYTH: "Try a sugar-free diet—cancer feeds on sugar." "Try eating only alkaline foods—cancers like to live in acid environments." "I swear by my juice cleanse. It literally purified my body and helped me fight off cancer better."

As discussed, there is currently *no* proven link between any specific dietary component and breast cancer. Yet this doesn't stop the news of faddy "cancer prevention" diets from making headlines in the press on a regular basis—and circulating among the wider population as a result. Many women turn to extreme dietary habits as a way of seeking control, assuming that cutting out purported cancer-promoting items will lead to better outcomes. From a medical perspective, these types of extreme diets are rarely advisable. Furthermore, these regimens are rarely sustainable. While it's a great idea to eat a balanced, plant-based diet with lots of fresh fruits and veggies and fewer highly processed foods packed with sugar and salt, there's no need to eliminate foods based on their alleged "cancer-causing" properties. Such regimens are usually not based on sound principles of overall health, so the best advice is to proceed with caution.

When it comes to sugar, yes, cancer does feed on sugar, but so do normal cells! In fact, all cells do. And guess what: *anything* you eat (protein, carbohydrate, fat) gets converted to sugar so cells can use it. So eating a diet composed of nothing but protein will not prevent cells in your body, good or bad, from seeing any sugar. And you cannot "starve" your cancer by depriving yourself of dietary sugar. The benefit of eating a healthy diet is that the sugar in these healthy foods comes with lots of good stuff too, like vitamins and minerals. Again, eating an overall healthy diet comprised of lots of fresh fruits and vegetables, lean meats, and whole grains, along with controlling your weight and minimizing alcohol intake, are your best bets for a good outcome, both for breast cancer and for your overall long-term health.

THE TAKEAWAY

- The only two lifestyle factors that are known to increase breast cancer risk and recurrence are obesity and heavy alcohol intake.
- Don't make yourself crazy with extreme health regimens or fads: a normal healthy diet, regular exercise, and not smoking are the factors that you control that will give you the best possible outcome for breast cancer and your long-term health.

CHAPTER 14

Alternative and Complementary Medicine

where do they fit in?

Lisa was a forty-seven-year-old mother of two when she had a mammogram and biopsy showing early cancer (DCIS). One of the first things Lisa said to me was, "I hope you're supportive of me taking an alternative medicine approach."

It turned out that Lisa had already been to see an internist, a holistic provider, *and* a herbalist, who had recommended that she start to take numerous supplements in the hope that this would build her immune system, begin to fight the cancer, and prepare her for her upcoming surgery.

I explained that if she was using the word "alternative" to mean simply taking her herbal treatments *instead of* standard interventions, then no, I would not be supportive. Those of us who are in the trenches fighting against cancer every day naturally become concerned when a patient is looking for another way to treat cancer outside of the mainstream treatments—surgery, medicine, radiation—that we know work. Most alternative treatments have yet to be extensively tested, so there are lots of unknowns with regard to toxicities and side effects, especially when combined with other treatments. However, if Lisa meant "complementary medicine"—which means taking other treatments *in addition to* the standard approach—then yes, I was supportive.

Complementary medicine (also called integrative medicine) has definitely increased in popularity, with many patients incorporating holistic and non-mainstream approaches into their overall care. My caveat with Lisa was that her different doctors—her surgeon, oncologist, internist, holistic provider, and herbalist—needed to be on the same page, so that we could make her aware of any treatments that competed with each other or exacerbated the toxic effect of another.

Lisa agreed to this approach. Together we examined every item on the list of supplements she was already taking. I told her I did have a concern about an "immune booster" given to her by her herbalist. The booster came in the form of a tablet taken by mouth, which means it goes into the stomach, gets absorbed into the bloodstream, and circulates throughout the body. I pointed out that when we put things in our bodies, we don't get to pick and choose where they end up. What if the "immune booster" was taken up by the cancer, which then used it to grow and become stronger? Lisa's jaw dropped when I brought this up. She had never thought of it that way.

In particular, it's important to carefully evaluate therapies that are ingested. Some supplements can actually undermine or adversely affect the standard medications you may be taking to treat your cancer. For example, certain herbs or mushrooms can have significant effects on the liver, and when these are taken in concert with certain chemotherapy agents—some of which are also metabolized by the liver—significant liver toxicity could result. So it takes expertise to decide what is safe to take and what isn't in combination with conventional medications.

The differences between complementary and alternative medicine

While alternative medicine implies using modalities outside of mainstream treatment options as *alternatives* to mainstream modalities, complementary medicine is a different story. By definition, "complementary" implies that treatments or therapies are given in concert with—and not in lieu of—standard regimens. Most modern major cancer centers have burgeoning complementary or integrative medicine departments with doctors who are serious about evaluating the effects of their therapies and optimizing combined treatments. Often these complementary treatments won't involve ingesting anything that could potentially compete with or cancel out the important treatments patients are taking. Rather, they focus on acupuncture, meditation, massage, and various therapies that can reduce stress and other side effects related to standard treatments. For example, new studies have shown that acupuncture may be able to reduce hot flashes, an unwanted side effect of some breast cancer medicine. Massage, yoga, hypnosis, and meditation all have potential complementary roles in the care of the cancer patient, and are implemented and widely promoted in most major cancer centers.

Rigorous testing: the fundamental difference between conventional and alternative medicine

Treatments that are standard for breast cancer today such as lumpectomy and chemotherapy have become standard only after years of skepticism, rigorous testing, and analysis. Good clinical trials are extremely difficult to conduct. They are expensive, costing millions of dollars to pay for personnel, data monitoring, and the actual treatment or drug that is being offered in the trial (since most patients participating in the trial are not charged for their treatment). Trials are time-consuming, and for a doctor, running a trial can absorb the better part of his or her career. And of course there is the amazing population of patients. People who agree to participate, whether for their own good or that of future generations, help make a great contribution to knowledge, science, and progress toward a better chance of cure for all. It can often take years just to organize and start a trial. And in order to accrue enough patients, many trials are conducted in multiple medical centers, treating patients from different centers all over the country and even the world, which is a huge organizational effort. (For more on research and clinical trials, see chapter 11.)

For example, before the 1970s, women only had mastectomies. With the advent of mammography, which detected cancers that are smaller, the concept of doing smaller surgery was conceived, but this was not just haphazardly implemented. Trials were performed in different countries in which women were randomly assigned to undergo mastectomy or lumpectomy coupled with radiation. The data from these trials was painstakingly analyzed to make sure that one group was similar to the other in terms of age, tumor size, lymph node status, and other variables. When the results ultimately showed no difference in survival, it formed the basis for what we now know as modern breast cancer surgery options: mastectomy or lumpectomy with radiation. So lumpectomy only became accepted as standard treatment after extensive and rigorous testing to make sure that it was as safe as mastectomy. And the data comparing lumpectomy with radiation and mastectomy has been revisited and reanalyzed numerous times since the study was originally reported over thirty years ago to verify that long-term outcomes continue to be excellent and equivalent.

Very few alternative regimens have been subjected to this same level of scrutiny, and it's rare that the alternative agent is pitted against the standard treatment in a thorough and rigorous trial. Yet this is truly the only way to objectively evaluate the effectiveness of a treatment. It's also good to know that alternative treatments tend to be attractive to patients when they run out of standard options or have a type of cancer for which there aren't many good options for treatment to begin with. But with breast cancer there are many treatments that have been well studied in large numbers of patients and are *known to work*. So selecting alternative treatments usually means opting for a course that is wholly unproven over treatments with proven track records. Of course, not all breast cancer treatments work in all cases. But choosing to take something alternative that has not been adequately evaluated *at all* over a treatment that is known to work for most women really doesn't make sense.

When concern for the side effects of conventional medicine leads one to consider alternative therapies instead

People often seek out alternative regimens because they are nervous about the known and unwanted side effects that come with standard treatments. But just because something is promoted as "natural" or "holistic" does not make it any safer or freer of side effects than something else that is synthetic or manufactured. There are many natural additives and ingredients that are quite toxic to the human body, and some in fact are poisonous. These are not safe and without side effects just because they are natural.

In fact, any agent that we ingest or inject—whether it's standard or alternative—may have some kind of side effect. For example, I had one patient who had a lumpectomy understanding that radiation and chemotherapy would be recommended afterward due to her large tumor size and lymph node involvement. Three months after her surgery, when she appeared in my office for a follow-up appointment, I was taken aback. Her skin had taken on a bizarre orange-yellow tone; she was almost glowing. She explained to me that instead of taking the recommended chemotherapy she had chosen to pursue an alternative treatment involving coffee enemas and megadoses of carrot juice (the culprit behind her bizarre skin tone). Her rationale was that she did not want the temporary side effects of nausea and hair loss from the chemo. And yet she was willing to walk around looking like a Martian for six months as a result of taking a treatment with no proven benefits! (And that's before you factor in the enemas, which, although "natural," could not have been particularly pleasant.)

If you do choose to go the alternative route, I would advise that you try to be as wary of the recommended alternative treatments as you would be of any standard medication. If the alternative agents are powerful enough to treat cancer, they will definitely have some side effects of their own. And conversely, if they have zero potential side effects, it's possible that they are no better than a placebo. If you are interested in incorporating integrative medicine approaches into your care, the Society for Integrative Oncology and its website (listed in the online resources section) are good resources for evidence-based information.

To take or not to take supplements

There is no evidence that most supplements have any effect, positive or negative, on the development or recurrence of breast cancer. Vendors can make all kinds of claims, and so can individuals. Your friend may swear that green tea extract prevented her breast cancer from coming back, but that doesn't mean it's been scientifically proven that green tea extract is effective or that her breast cancer wouldn't have been effectively treated without it. And remember, as with Lisa, my patient in the beginning of this chapter, any supplement that you ingest while you are fighting cancer that is purported to have a positive effect on your body and its cells may be exerting its positive effect for your cancer cells.

Supplements and vitamins are a multibillion-dollar industry in the United States. Even patients who are otherwise healthy and generally averse to taking medicine will come into my office with a long list of supplements that they have been taking for years: vitamins A through Z, gingko biloba, coenzyme Q, chondroitin, fish oils, omega-3 fatty acids, echinacea, shark cartilage . . . the list goes on and on. It's worth keeping in mind that most alternative treatments and their dosing are totally unregulated, and therefore the producers of these products are not obligated to adhere to any specific standards regarding potency or even to prove effectiveness. For example, if you look at "shark cartilage" tablets from ten different sources, the actual amount of shark cartilage in each tablet varies from almost nothing to quite high. And there is no regulatory body that reviews these products and makes sure that the amount of shark cartilage in each tablet is appropriate before it can be marketed. In part this is because there is no dose of shark cartilage that has been proven to be effective and there is no dosage that has proven to be safe. So the amount to take and the amount you are actually receiving in each tablet are completely arbitrary. The severity of the problem related to lack of oversight in the supplement industry was recently brought to light when the New York attorney general accused four major retail chains of selling "fraudulent and potentially dangerous herbal supplements and demanded that they remove the products from their shelves" (*The New York Times,* February 3, 2015). In their investigation, four out of five supplements tested contained *none* of the agents they purportedly contained: the ginkgo biloba contained powdered radish, wheat, and houseplants! These agents are hardly choice ingredients for treating cancer (or any other ailment, for that matter), and can actually contain dangerous toxins and cause severe allergic reactions to the contents that are not even listed on the label.

Taking supplements that may or may not even contain the agent they are reported to contain, in amounts that cannot be quantified, is not exactly the most precise or desirable way to treat a cancer.

At least conventional medications have to go through FDA approval and rigorous testing in clinical trials—and as a result, much is known about the benefits and side effects, both short-term and long-term. But supplements almost never go through scientific testing. (They're also expensive: you can easily spend hundreds of dollars for a mere one-month supply.)

I never really understood why so many women who are skeptical of medications and reluctant to take them unless absolutely necessary are so willing to take additives about which little if anything is really known. Again, my recommendation when it comes to supplements, additives, and other miracle cures—especially the expensive ones—is that you be at least as skeptical and as inquisitive as you would be about *any* medicine. And be particularly wary of the products that a doctor may be promoting and selling out of his or her own office or from which he or she will otherwise financially benefit. Then if you end up going ahead with the recommended course, make sure *all* your doctors know about everything you are taking.

The exception to the rule: vitamin D and calcium

There is no question that with rigorous testing, there is some possibility that supplements, vitamins, and other additives could be found to play a role in cancer prevention and recurrence. For example, there is good data to suggest that there may be a role for supplementing vitamin D and calcium in your diet *if* these are deficient. Vitamin D and calcium are both important to bone health and strength, especially for postmenopausal women, and there is some evidence that women who are deficient in vitamin D may have an increased risk of their cancer recurring. This has led many health care professionals to recommend testing for vitamin D levels and supplementation for those who are deficient. These recommendations are made based on actual information and data.

Spirituality and religion: for many, the best complementary medicine

For many people, religion and spirituality play central roles in their everyday lives. When a patient goes through a life-changing event such as a breast cancer diagnosis, spirituality and religious beliefs can play an important part in the coping process and thus can have an integral role in your overall care.

Religion, faith, and spirituality can be important sources of comfort and strength, and can take many forms. Whether your particular leanings involve organized religion and a specific religious community or just a belief in a guiding force or a sense that you are being protected, your faith can serve as a great source of hope and optimism that's completely complementary to your medical treatments.

As a surgeon, I have been asked to do everything from standing in the middle of a family prayer circle with a patient before walking into the operating room with her to tucking a meaningful prayer written on a piece of paper under the patient's pillow in the OR. Once a priest blessed my hands and poured holy water on them before surgery (even though he knew I still had to scrub afterward). When patients tell me they say prayers for me and my family, I am always moved: they want me to be protected, just as, they believe, I have played a small role in protecting them. In my personal religious community, part of our religious service involves a prayer for healing. We are asked to stand and recite this prayer together if anyone we know is in need of healing, and I always do. Any type of spiritual connection that helps a person feel better, more confident, and optimistic about her outcome works for me.

THE TAKEAWAY

- When it comes to supplements and other alternative treatments, make sure your doctors are all on the same page regarding anything you are taking before, during, and after cancer treatment.
- Complementary treatments such as acupuncture, meditation, and massage can help alleviate stress and some side effects of conventional treatments.
- Ingested substances can "feed" bad cells as easily as they can feed good cells.
- Be as skeptical about alternative remedies as you are about standard, conventional treatments.

CHAPTER 15

Cancer Is a Family Affair . . .

and what are those genes that everyone keeps talking about?

M y patient Christina is one of three sisters. After she was diagnosed with breast cancer at age thirty-seven—and successfully treated—her older sister, Jenna, joined our breast cancer high-risk program. I now see Jenna in my office every six months, and she has mammograms once a year every summer and MRIs once a year every winter. The third sister, Valerie, is only twenty-five and is reluctant to start screening for breast cancer at such a young age, although she too will likely join our program in the next few years. As these sisters know, when one person in a family is diagnosed, it can have a domino effect, raising risk (and anxiety) for the other female family members.

My newly diagnosed patients are usually—and understandably— extremely anxious about the possibility of an increased risk for their daughters, sisters, and mothers. The good news is that when one person in a family is diagnosed, the increased risk to other female family members is not always as high as you might think. For instance, a single family member diagnosed with breast cancer at the age of seventy may not increase her daughter's risk by very much overall. However, if multiple relatives are diagnosed, particularly at young ages, this could increase their relatives' risk to a greater extent. Thankfully, in this day and age, once we've established an increased risk, we can screen women with greater frequency and vigilance so that if they do develop the disease we have the best chance of detecting it early, leading to the best chance for cure. We can also suggest genetic testing if appropriate, to determine whether there is a genetic predisposition in the family.

Genetic predisposition: BRCA-1 and BRCA-2

Most of my patients have read or heard something about the BRCA-1 and BRCA-2 genes and have questions about whether they may be affected. BRCA-1 and BRCA-2 are genes that everyone has, but when these genes are mutated or faulty they lead to a very high risk of developing both breast and ovarian cancers, while also raising the risk for other cancers to a lesser degree (such as pancreatic cancer and prostate cancer, as well as male breast cancer for those affected by BRCA-2). In order to be tested for the BRCA gene mutation you will need to give a blood or saliva sample so that DNA can be analyzed. Results usually take between ten days and three weeks.

If it is determined that you do have the mutation, then your risk of developing breast cancer can be as high as 80 to 90 percent, and your risk of developing ovarian cancer can vary from 20 to 40 percent. For women who have already been diagnosed with breast cancer and who are then tested and found to have a BRCA mutation, their risk of developing a *second* breast cancer, either in the same breast or in the opposite breast, can be quite high: up to 50 percent. If this is the case for you, then you may consider more extensive surgery, such as removing both breasts, just to avoid the development of future breast cancers. (See chapter 6 for more on factors influencing surgical decision making.)

Women who are BRCA mutation carriers frequently develop cancer at much younger ages, commonly in their thirties and forties. For women who do carry the gene, these numbers are obviously a cause for concern: there is no one at higher risk for breast cancer than women who have BRCA mutations. Meanwhile, men in the family who carry the gene are at risk for developing prostate, pancreatic, and male breast cancer, but these risks are much lower (for example, the male breast cancer risk is approximately 10 percent for men with BRCA-2 mutations).

MYTH: "If you have a family history of breast cancer, you must have the BRCA-gene."

The BRCA-1 and BRCA-2 mutations are actually rare, and they are responsible for a very small proportion of breast cancers overall. Only approximately two of every thousand women (or 0.2 percent of the general population) is likely to carry the gene. Even among families with a history of breast and/or ovarian cancer, only a minority of these cases will be caused by BRCA mutations. But because genes often cluster in different ways among people of different ethnicities, the prevalence of a given problematic gene is often higher among specific groups of people. So, for example, among the Ashkenazi Jewish population—Jewish people whose ancestors come from Europe—the BRCA mutation is much more common and is found in approximately 2 percent of the population (or one in forty women). As a result, many women who are Ashkenazi Jewish do get tested, especially if they have a family history of breast or ovarian cancer, or after being diagnosed with breast or ovarian cancer themselves.

When you should—and shouldn't—consider getting tested

"You've been diagnosed with breast cancer. You need to get tested for the BRCA gene."

This is something that women with breast cancer are told by well-meaning friends and family members all the time. It's a very common misconception that every woman with a breast cancer diagnosis herself or in her family needs to get tested for the mutation. However, for women who are postmenopausal, with no family history of breast cancer, and not Ashkenazi Jewish—in other words, the vast majority of women diagnosed—there's a very low likelihood of testing positive; in fact, fewer than 10 percent of all breast cancer patients are found to have the BRCA gene mutation. Certainly you can discuss testing with your doctor, and asking can never be a bad thing, but it is not a given that every woman needs to get tested. In fact, for the majority, there is no need.

Most breast cancer specialists are quite familiar with BRCA gene testing and when it's appropriate to send patients for screening. In many cases, BRCA testing is recommended once a woman has been diagnosed with cancer and we are concerned that she may have the genetic mutation. If she tests positive, then other close family members, both male and female, may also want to get tested—even if they are healthy—as each of her children or siblings has a fifty-fifty chance of also having inherited the gene.

Here are the red-flag scenarios where we're most likely to recommend BRCA testing:

1. Women from families with two premenopausal first-degree relatives with breast cancer. A first-degree relative is a mother, daughter, or sister.
2. Women with a personal or family history of both breast and ovarian cancer.
3. Women with family histories that include male breast cancer.
4. Any woman diagnosed with breast cancer at a young age (some use forty as a cutoff, some use fifty) regardless of her family history.
5. Any woman who is Ashkenazi Jewish and diagnosed with breast cancer at any age.
6. Any woman diagnosed with cancer in both breasts, especially if the first cancer was diagnosed before age fifty.
7. Any woman diagnosed with triple negative breast cancer especially at a young age (because of its strong association with BRCA-1).
8. Any woman diagnosed with two separate breast cancers (typically bilateral breast cancer).
9. Extenuating circumstances. There are many situations that don't meet standard testing criteria but in which genetic testing should nevertheless at least be discussed and considered individually. What does a woman with breast cancer do if she was adopted and has no idea about her biological family's medical history? Or what if a woman with breast cancer is an only child and her mother died at a young age of other causes? How would she know if she actually had a family history when there are very few family members at all? In such cases where little or nothing is

known about family history, we often discuss options for testing and what it might mean. Also, families with a disproportionate amount of very rare cancer among the relatives may also be recommended for testing.

Again, it's worth noting that most women do not fall into any of these nine red-flag categories. Seventy-five percent of women diagnosed with breast cancer are older than fifty, 80 to 90 percent have no family history, and only a very small percentage of the population is Ashkenazi Jewish. Recently, there have been initiatives proposed to offer and perform genetic testing on *entire* populations of women, regardless of personal or family history of breast cancer. The rationale behind this vision is that identifying someone who is an unsuspected BRCA mutation carrier could lead to action that prevents cancer, the need for treatment, and the risk of mortality related to it. Many in our field believe that a BRCA mutation carrier who actually develops breast cancer represents a failure, because it could potentially have been prevented had we known about her genetic status. Interest in this type of initiative has been proposed mainly for the Ashkenazi Jewish population specifically, where one in every forty women (and men) will test positive. The bottom line is that, regardless of your ethnic background or family history, it's completely reasonable to discuss the appropriateness of BRCA testing with your doctor, especially if you feel you fit into any of the categories above.

Genetic counseling

While many doctors can order the BRCA test themselves, sending you to a genetic counselor for discussion and testing is the preferred approach, and in some cases this extra consultation is required in order to have your insurer pay for the testing. Most major medical centers and almost all breast cancer programs have genetic counseling services. Genetic counselors are trained to ask questions about your family relationships and medical history that might help determine your need for the test. Family histories can be complicated and misleading, especially in families with small numbers of women, but genetic counselors have expertise and training in identifying any red flags.

For example, many people—even some doctors—don't realize that the gene mutation can be handed down through both the mother's *and* the father's side of the family. So the genetic counselor will ask detailed questions about both the maternal and paternal sides of your family. While there is a slightly higher risk of developing other cancers associated with BRCA-1 and BRCA-2—and male breast cancer is associated with BRCA-2 (see chapter 16 on male breast cancer)—the gene usually does not rear its ugly head in men, and so it can be passed down silently through generations of men before affecting any female offspring.

Also important to know is that there are other, rare genetic syndromes that are associated with increased risk of breast cancer. Li-Fraumeni syndrome involves the mutation of a gene called p53. When p53 is mutated it is associated with a variety of different cancers, including sarcomas, brain tumors, leukemia, and, yes, breast cancer. Another, Lynch syndrome, is more frequently associated with colon and uterine cancers, but there is also an associated higher risk of breast cancer (albeit not as high as that seen with a BRCA mutation). And there are other rare genetic syndromes as well. Thankfully, these types of mutations affect only a very small proportion of the population. However, if rare cancers have disproportionately affected your family, then genetic counseling and testing will likely be recommended. Genetic counselors are trained to ask the appropriate questions that might tease out the possibility of a BRCA or other mutation, thereby helping define your and your family members' risks of developing disease.

BRCA testing when you *do* have breast cancer

For those who are at risk for the genetic mutation (see previously described criteria) and are newly diagnosed with breast cancer, testing is very important because it can play a key role in making decisions going forward.

What the BRCA test results mean for surgery:

1. If you have a breast cancer diagnosis and you're found to be *negative* for the BRCA mutation (you don't have it), then we know that the risk of cancer coming back in the same breast is likely

low. In addition, the risk of developing a new cancer on the other side is quite low as well, usually less than 5 percent. So a lumpectomy is very likely to be a reasonable option for you even if you do have a family history of breast cancer.

2. If you have a breast cancer diagnosis and you're found to be *positive* for the gene mutation (you do have it), then the risk of having the cancer come back in the same breast is high, perhaps 30 percent, and the risk for a new cancer developing in the other breast is significantly higher as well, up to 50 percent. This leads many women to consider having more extensive surgery, such as bilateral mastectomy, to reduce the high likelihood of a second cancer occurring. The caveat to this is that some women who do have the gene mutation are diagnosed with breast cancer later in life than would be expected with BRCA-associated cancers, which usually occur in a woman's thirties or forties. There is some evidence that if you are BRCA positive and diagnosed with your first breast cancer after the age of fifty your likelihood of recurrence may be lower than usually expected, and thus lumpectomy may be reasonable.

Although test results can take anywhere from ten days to three weeks to come through, many women will choose to wait for them to come back before making a final decision regarding surgery. In the ideal scenario, the blood or saliva specimen is sent off right away after diagnosis, so that surgery is not unnecessarily delayed.

NEED TO KNOW

Some women, especially those with a family history of breast cancer, will opt to have more extensive surgery regardless of their results from genetic testing. Many of my patients with breast cancer are adamant that they want a bilateral mastectomy, and for them, waiting for the results won't change their minds or their choice. But for other women, the choice may not be as clear-cut. If you fall into this second camp, where genetic results could help you make the decision about the kind of surgery you're going to have, it's important to know that waiting the few weeks for genetic testing results before making your decision is not dangerous and will *not* jeopardize your chance for cure.

A WORD TO THE WISE

Most women who test positive for the BRCA mutation tend to opt for mastectomy. For the woman who has a BRCA mutation and who wants to go ahead anyway with lumpectomy and radiation, there is a caveat. It's important to keep in mind that if the cancer comes back and mastectomy becomes necessary down the line, the options for reconstruction may be compromised due to the effects of radiation on the skin (for more about this, go to chapter 10). In addition, treatment options may not be as extensive the second time around. Bottom line: when you have a known higher risk of recurrence, you need to discuss this with your doctor and consider your options very carefully.

BRCA testing when you *don't* have breast cancer

The most common scenario in which a woman *without* breast cancer is tested for the BRCA gene is when her close family member—commonly a mother or a sister—develops breast cancer and is found to have the genetic mutation. When that happens, all first-degree family members each have a fifty-fifty chance of having inherited the gene—and so genetic testing is highly recommended.

If you do not have a breast cancer diagnosis but are concerned about carrying the gene, your doctor should first determine if a close family member who has had breast or ovarian cancer has been tested and found to be positive for BRCA-1 or BRCA-2. If a relative *with* breast cancer has already been tested and does *not* carry the gene, there is usually no reason to test you.

In some cases, a woman might come to my office with a strong history of breast and ovarian cancer in her family, and even though no one in her family who had cancer has been tested, we might still go ahead with the test. This is because BRCA testing was first introduced in the mid-1990s, and so for some women, their family members with the disease may have already passed away without having been tested.

If you are a woman *without* breast cancer who is concerned about carrying the BRCA gene and wants to get tested, the testing can proceed with less time pressure, as there is no rush to get results to better plan for cancer surgery. The results are still important, however, because they will affect your screening and options going forward. We usually do not test young women without breast cancer before the age of approximately twenty to twenty-five, which is the approximate age when developing breast cancer becomes a realistic possibility, and also when young women can start to understand their risks and make serious decisions about these risks. Before then, the risk of getting breast cancer is quite low even in those who test positive for the gene.

What the test results will mean for your screening regimen:

1. If you're found to be negative for the gene mutation, then you can continue with a regular screening regimen: mammograms annually after the age of forty, or ten years younger than when your youngest relative was diagnosed. Even if you are BRCA negative, you may still receive a recommendation to undergo additional imaging studies, such as ultrasounds and MRIs, depending on your actual risk level. (For more on screening regimens in high-risk patients and determining risk, see chapter 1.)

2. If you're found to be positive for the BRCA mutation, then your risk of developing breast cancer in the future is extremely high, possibly approaching 80 to 90 percent. You are also more likely to develop your cancer before the age of forty when screening is recommended to start for the general population. Importantly, the age at which you might develop breast or ovarian cancer cannot be known or predicted, even by looking at the history of other family members and their ages at diagnosis. As a result, the usual recommendation for women who test positive for the gene is to initiate screening early and with greater rigor and frequency. Your doctor will most likely recommend you start annual mammograms and MRIs beginning at age twenty-five. The tests can

be performed together, or split up so you are getting a test every six months. Breast examinations are also important to detect cancers that might develop between imaging tests, and are usually recommended two to four times a year.

Risk-reducing mastectomies

Risk-reducing mastectomy for BRCA mutation carriers has been in the news of late, with various celebrities going public with their decision to reduce cancer risk by removing both breasts (Angelina Jolie being the most prominent example). Given the extremely high risk of developing breast cancer for women with the BRCA gene mutation, the rigorous screening regimen required, and the anxiety associated with so many tests and the biopsies they engender, it's not surprising that many people with BRCA mutations seek other options.

If you are a sister, daughter, or even a mother of a breast or ovarian cancer patient who has been tested and discovered to have the gene, then bilateral prophylactic or "risk-reducing" mastectomy (removing both breasts) is certainly an option for you. Removing the ovaries is usually also recommended in women near age forty and/or when childbearing is completed, as there is really no effective screening for ovarian cancer, leading to late-stage ovarian cancer diagnosis for most women who develop the disease.

Needless to say, the decision to undergo risk-reducing surgery is a very personal choice. By definition this type of surgery is elective, and so the decision making process doesn't only involve deciding yes or no; it also involves when. For example, do you wait until after childbearing is completed so you can breastfeed? Or do you do it before you have children so that you don't have to experience the fear and anxiety of cancer developing while your breasts grow and change, as they inevitably will during pregnancy? As with many aspects of decision making around breast cancer, there is no one-size-fits-all choice. The perfect timing for one woman may be too soon or too late for another. Most women arrive at the decision over time, not immediately and impulsively. My advice is to talk beforehand with a breast surgeon and a plastic surgeon (most women who undergo risk-reducing mastectomy do opt for reconstruction), and of course undergo appropriate screening and examination to make sure there is nothing currently concerning.

A WORD TO THE WISE

For optimal results, risk-reducing mastectomies should really be performed by a very experienced breast surgeon. An experienced surgeon will be committed to removing as much breast tissue as possible, as any remaining breast tissue or cells could potentially develop cancer. For more on finding the right surgeon, go to chapter 4.

When BRCA is not a factor

Deborah is a young woman who felt a lump in her breast. Her mother had been diagnosed with breast cancer at age forty-nine. She visited her gynecologist, who reassured her that it was almost certainly a benign lump or cyst, related to cyclical hormonal changes. She advised her to wait one month and come back. One month later the mass was still there, not significantly changed, and Deborah's doctor sent her for a sonogram to prove to her that it was a cyst. It wasn't. After a sonogram, a mammogram, and two biopsies, Deborah came to my office with a diagnosis of breast cancer at age twenty-three.

There are definitely those families where, one by one, the women are stricken with breast cancer, many at very young ages. These family members' medical histories may give the impression that the BRCA gene is the culprit, yet one by one, family members are tested, and no one in the family is found to have BRCA or any other identifiable genetic mutation. We see families like this all the time, where we *know* there is some kind of genetic predisposition; it's just that we can't test for it. Members of these families are among the toughest to counsel. At least with the BRCA mutation carriers we have some clear-cut information regarding the known risks, and women can have specific information that's useful when they're making decisions about surgery, treatment, and screening. For women who have strong family histories but aren't mutation carriers, we don't have the same degree of information regarding their future risk, and this can be a significant source of anxiety for both patients and their doctors. Our hope is that in the future, other types of testing and understanding can become available so that we can better serve these families.

THE TAKEAWAY

- Not everyone who is diagnosed with breast cancer or who has breast cancer in the family needs to get genetic testing. Your doctor can help you decide whether testing is appropriate for you.
- If you have a BRCA mutation and breast cancer, you may decide to opt for bilateral mastectomies; if you have a lumpectomy, there is a good chance you will be dealing with breast cancer again.
- Currently, risk-reducing mastectomy is the only effective way to prevent breast cancer for BRCA mutation carriers. But the decision to have this type of surgery is personal and elective.

CHAPTER 16

Yes, Men Can Get Breast Cancer Too

less information, but also less information overload

Male breast cancer is extremely rare. There are only about 2,500 cases diagnosed in the United States each year (compared to the 300,000 women who are diagnosed with breast cancer during the same period). As a result, there's very little awareness among the general public about this issue. And when a man is diagnosed with breast cancer, it's generally true to say he's caught completely off guard.

I can remember one patient, Rob, who came to me on his doctor's recommendation after finding a lump under his right nipple. We did a mammogram and ultrasound, then two needle biopsies that confirmed breast cancer both in the lump behind the nipple and under his armpit in a lymph node. Rob was in his fifties, but unlike many women the same age, he hadn't been thinking about breast cancer—and he'd certainly never had a mammogram before! The word "shock" can't begin to describe Rob's reaction when he learned that this was his diagnosis. Not surprisingly, he had a barrage of questions, the first of which was "Why have I gotten a female cancer? I didn't even know this could happen to men!" I reassured him that male breast cancer is *not* a female cancer. The disease is different in men and has completely different ramifications physically, mentally, and emotionally.

MYTH: "Male breast cancer is more life-threatening than female breast cancer because it's rarer."

Breast cancer is *absolutely* as treatable and curable in men, and survival rates are basically the same as with women at comparable stages of disease. So we have plenty of room for optimism. But male breast cancer is usually detected later in men than it is with women because they aren't usually screened with mammograms, and because of decreased awareness.

Rob had initially assumed that the lump under his nipple was a skin cyst, and he had simply waited for it to disappear. Because he had delayed for many months before seeing a doctor, his cancer had already spread to the lymph nodes.

For his part, Rob handled his diagnosis and treatment beautifully. He did say it was hard for many of his male friends, who, while trying to be supportive, had not known other men with breast cancer before and often didn't know what to say. He once darkly joked with me that most of his male friends were reaching the age where they were starting to worry and talk about prostate cancer so much that *his* diagnosis with breast cancer had actually become an interesting diversion. Rob didn't seem to experience the same level of information overload and bombardment with suggestions and recommendations from others that many female patients do, perhaps because male breast cancer is so rare. This has its advantages, but also has its disadvantages: few to bond and commiserate with, and support groups filled exclusively with women. As with many individuals who are diagnosed with a rare cancer, Rob made his own way, with the support of his doctors and his family and close friends.

Causes

We don't know nearly as much about breast cancer in men as we do about breast cancer in women, but there are risk factors that have been identified for male breast cancer. These include a variety of rare chromosomal abnormalities, as well as increased estrogen exposure and genetic predisposition, especially with the BRCA-2 gene, which is associated with an increased breast cancer risk to around 10 percent for men (for more on BRCA-2, go to chapter 15). Gynecomastia, or the male breast enlargement that is typical in older or heavier men, is *not* a risk factor for developing breast cancer.

Detection and diagnosis

Most cases of male breast cancer are found after the patient himself detects some kind of abnormality, usually a lump directly under the nipple. The reason for this is that almost all male breast cancers originate in the ducts of the breast, and most of the ducts in the male breast are directly behind the nipple. Because the cancer is often so close in proximity to the nipple it can be associated with visible nipple changes such as inversion, bleeding, or discharge, any of which may be the first sign that something is wrong. Oftentimes men will first notice a lump under their arm because the cancer has already spread to the lymph nodes, and the patient hasn't realized that there was a lump or change in the breast in the first place.

As with female breast cancer, a needle biopsy is the best way to make a diagnosis. Most commonly, an ultrasound can identify the mass and then a needle is directed to the center of the suspicious area. The snippets of tissue that are removed can be analyzed under the microscope to make a definitive diagnosis. Surgical biopsies, which involve a trip to the operating room to make an incision so that a portion of the mass can be removed, should be reserved for cases where the needle biopsy could not be done but where there is still a concern (see chapter 2 for more on needle biopsies versus surgical biopsies).

Treatment

With so few cases of male breast cancer each year, it's impossible to perform randomized trials to know specifically which treatments work best for male breast cancer, and so treatment options are essentially extrapolated from those that work for women. Like the treatment of breast cancer in women, most male breast cancer treatment starts with surgery and progresses through medical treatment (chemotherapy and hormonal treatment) if needed. Radiation is also given if needed.

Even among specialists, there are very few surgeons, medical oncologists, or radiation oncologists and very few centers treating more than a few cases of breast cancer in men per year—which is why it's essential for men to be treated at a center known for excellence. If you don't live near one of these, you should definitely consider traveling for your treatment. As an additional benefit, most advanced breast centers are well set up to accommodate male patients in a private, gender-neutral way so men can get through their experience without the pink examination robes and ribbons, and with their dignity intact.

Surgery

Breast cancer surgery and decision making for men are very different than they are for women.

Most male breasts are relatively small, and therefore lumpectomy—where only the lump and the surrounding tissue are removed—is not an option. Instead, mastectomy is the standard surgery recommended for male breast cancer. For men, as with women, mastectomy means removing all the breast tissue up to the clavicle, down to the abdomen, to the sternum in the center and across to the latissimus dorsi muscle under the arm. A standard male mastectomy includes removal of the nipple and areolar complex (surrounding darker-colored skin), since in most male breast cancer cases, the cancer is near or virtually inseparable from the nipple.

We don't tend to perform breast reconstruction for men, as in most cases—especially for patients with hairy chests—the minimal asymmetry from the slightly flatter chest wall, the mastectomy scar, and the lack of nipple is barely visible. Occasionally a tattoo of the nipple can re-create it over the mastectomy scar, but this isn't very commonly done or requested.

Lymph nodes

As with female breast cancer, when male breast cancer spreads it most commonly goes first to the lymph nodes under the arm. (See chapter 5 for a full explanation of the lymph nodes and their function.) Determining lymph node status in male breast cancer is as critically important for management as it is in women. Even when lymph nodes feel normal on exam and there is no obvious spread, we need to check them at surgery to find out for sure. Sentinel node biopsy—which involves injecting dye into the breast tissue that then travels to a few select nodes under the arm—is the standard procedure for checking lymph node status in women, and is definitely recommended in men. I am proud to say that along with my colleagues at the time at Memorial Sloan-Kettering, I was one of the first to demonstrate that sentinel node biopsy is just as accurate for checking lymph nodes in male breast cancer patients as it is for females. Sentinel node biopsy is performed in surgery at the same time as mastectomy, usually through the same incision. And when sentinel nodes are tested and found to be normal (negative), additional node removal—a much larger procedure associated with greater risk of complications—is not necessary.

For many cases of male breast cancer, however, the cancer has already spread to the lymph nodes by the time we find it. Sometimes the surgeon can feel an enlarged, suspicious node on examination, and sometimes an imaging study, either a mammogram or ultrasound, is an indicator. A needle biopsy done of the node or nodes that are suspicious can tell us about node spread before any surgery is done, and help to guide the operative procedure as a result. Specifically, if nodes are proven to have cancer *before* surgery, sentinel node biopsy is no longer necessary, as the node status has already been determined. For these cases where nodes are known to have cancer, removal of all the nodes, or axillary dissection, is the standard procedure. With axillary dissection the main risk is lymphedema, which is swelling of the arm due to lymph fluid, normally filtered by lymph nodes, accumulating in the arm due to severed outflow pathways. Early mobilization and strengthening can reduce this risk. Numbness, other side effects, and restrictions can also result from axillary dissection. (See chapter 5 for more information on axillary dissection and chapter 12 for more information on recovery from this operation.)

TREATMENT AFTER SURGERY

Chemotherapy

As with women, chemotherapy is often recommended for men with larger tumors and positive nodes. In general, chemotherapy is given in treatment cycles, every two to three weeks, using the same agents that are recommended for women. Each cycle involves intravenous infusion of one or more drugs over a few hours. The side effects of chemotherapy can be the same in men as they are for women—although when it comes to hair loss, most of my male patients shave their heads and go bald; almost none get a wig. (See chapter 9 for more on chemotherapy treatment and its side effects.)

Endocrine therapy

Over 90 percent of male breast cancers are hormone receptor positive, meaning that estrogen and progesterone fuel the growth and spread of their cancer. This is in contrast to breast cancer in women, where approximately 60 to 70 percent of cases are hormonally responsive. As a result, most men are advised to take an anti-hormonal agent as part of their treatment. Tamoxifen, given as a pill, is usually recommended to be taken for at least five years. When it comes to aromatase inhibitors, which are now the treatment of choice for postmenopausal women, there is less overall experience in using them for treatment in men. Side effects from these endocrine therapy agents, which affect hormonal levels in the body, are different for men than for women and can include hot flashes and decreased libido. Studies have shown that men are less likely to adhere to hormonal treatment than their female counterparts, which may be because they don't tolerate the side effects as well. However, most men do tolerate hormonal treatments well and complete treatment as recommended. (See chapter 9 for more on hormonal agents.)

Radiation

Because most men don't have lumpectomies, most men don't need radiation. But there are some criteria for giving radiation even after mastectomy. As with women, men with more advanced cancers, as indicated by a larger tumor or significant lymph node involvement, may be recommended for radiation as well. (See chapter 10 regarding indications for radiation after mastectomy.) Treatment involves receiving radiation beams to the chest wall and lymph node areas, usually for five minutes five days a week for six weeks. Side effects can be tanning and burning of the skin (similar to a bad sunburn), which is temporary; fatigue is common toward the end of the duration of treatment. The risk of lymphedema can be further increased when radiation is required on top of axillary dissection.

The BRCA factor

Most men diagnosed with male breast cancer should be tested for genetic predisposition, as the BRCA-2 mutation is found in approximately 10 percent of male breast cancer patients. And men who are known to carry the BRCA-2 mutation have a 10 percent risk of developing male breast cancer over their lifetimes. While a 10 percent risk does not seem high, it is about the same level of risk for developing breast cancer as the average woman over her lifetime, and as a result, screening with yearly mammogram is definitely recommended in this selected group of men. In addition, if you find out that you are BRCA-2 positive, this can also be helpful in screening for other cancers, and could be important for your children—both male and female—in determining whether they are at significantly higher risk for developing breast, ovarian, and other cancers. (See chapter 15 on BRCA mutations.)

The emotional impact

I always tell my male patients that there is no need to feel embarrassed or stigmatized in any way after a breast cancer diagnosis. However, it's only natural for most men to feel isolated. There is so little awareness of male breast cancer in the general community that telling others can be challenging and is usually met with shock and disbelief. Many men diagnosed with this rare disease are inspired to raise awareness, and I have seen many male patients who use their diagnosis as a springboard to do much good for their communities.

Unlike my female patients, who usually benefit from the community of fellow patients and survivors, most of the men I see tend to avoid joining support groups, as these are predominantly women only. Many of the issues that affect women going through breast cancer treatment simply aren't the same for men: rarely do men with breast cancer feel that the loss of a breast affects their attractiveness or self-image, and almost no men have to grapple with the process of reconstruction. However, it can still help to speak with others who have gone through treatment for cancer, whether it's breast cancer or another cancer. After all, any human being diagnosed with cancer thinks about survival and mortality, and everyone has to deal with both the physical and emotional side effects of both the disease and the treatment. What I've seen is that most men with breast cancer carve their own path, using their doctors, family members, and close friends as support.

THE TAKEAWAY

- Male breast cancer is rare and so needs to be treated at a center of excellence if at all possible.
- Male breast cancer is usually diagnosed as a mass, and at a later stage, because most men are not regularly screened.
- Treatment is similar to that for women, although lumpectomy is not usually an option for men.
- Survival for male breast cancer is the same as that for women, stage for stage. The fact that it is rare does not make it any more dangerous in terms of mortality.

CHAPTER 17

Breast Cancer During Pregnancy, and Pregnancy After Breast Cancer

both can happen

Most breast cancers are diagnosed in women age fifty and older. As a result, it's relatively uncommon for women to be diagnosed during their childbearing years. However, a small percentage of breast cancer cases are diagnosed in women in their twenties and thirties, which means being diagnosed with breast cancer while pregnant is absolutely possible. And for younger women who aren't pregnant yet but hope to become pregnant in the future, a breast cancer diagnosis and its treatment can strongly impact future fertility. While there is never a "good" time for *any* woman of *any* age to be diagnosed with breast cancer, its impact on younger age groups relative to plans for childbearing brings an added level of complexity: for women who are pregnant or hoping to become pregnant, breast cancer is never part of the plan.

Jessica is a thirty-six-year-old doctor. She and her husband of five years, who is also a doctor, held off on getting pregnant and having children knowing that the exhausting process of medical school and residency would be too much for the two of them while also worrying about the care of a child. Jessica had just finished her residency training and was in her first year in private practice when she noticed a lump in her left breast while taking a shower. She knew enough not to try to self-diagnose, and so she saw her gynecologist, who ordered a mammogram and ultrasound. The next day, Jessica went for her imaging studies and was met by a technologist who asked her the usual round of questions: "Any family history of breast cancer?" "No." "Any previous mammograms or biopsies?" "No." "Any chance you are pregnant?" Jessica started to answer "No," but then stopped herself, realizing she wasn't so sure. She had stopped taking her birth control pills a few months earlier, in the hope of getting pregnant, but assumed it would take a while. "You better do a pregnancy test," Jessica told the tech. A few minutes later, the radiologist came in to speak to Jessica. "Let's just start with an ultrasound, which is totally safe during pregnancy, just in case," she advised. On the ultrasound a two-centimeter irregular mass was found in the area that Jessica felt, and a needle biopsy was done. One hour later Jessica's pregnancy test came back: "You are pregnant," the radiologist told her. One day later Jessica's biopsy result came back: "And you have breast cancer." It was a heartbreaking time for Jessica, her husband, and her family, who had to make some extremely high-stakes decisions about her health, her growing fetus, *and* her future fertility.

There are many reasons why managing breast cancer during a woman's childbearing years can be more complicated and challenging than at any other time. Here are the key factors to know and understand when it comes to breast cancer, pregnancy, and fertility.

Breast cancer *during* pregnancy

Breast cancer during pregnancy is rare, occurring in approximately one in three thousand pregnancies; however, it has become more frequent given the increase in the number of women delaying childbearing (breast cancer becomes more common as we age). And while every breast cancer diagnosis is devastating, there is no doubt that it's earth-shattering if you're pregnant. Overnight, this joyful time in your life becomes fraught with seemingly impossible decisions about how to protect your own health while also protecting the health of your unborn child.

Diagnosis

Women diagnosed with breast cancer during pregnancy are more likely to have larger tumors, since normal changes to breast tissue during pregnancy can make it more difficult to notice a new or changing lump, thus delaying diagnosis. There is also a higher likelihood of spread to the lymph nodes, and therefore the requirement of additional, stronger treatment. This is not to say that treatment for breast cancer isn't possible or can't be successful during pregnancy—it absolutely can; it's just a more complicated process.

Mammograms and MRIs are not commonly done during pregnancy in order to protect the fetus from exposure to radiation (in the case of mammograms) or gadolinium (in the case of MRIs). But ultrasounds can definitely be done safely, and should be used without hesitation to investigate any new or enlarging lump. When necessary, a mammogram can be done during pregnancy with some shielding of the abdomen to reduce radiation exposure to the fetus.

Treatment

Making decisions about breast cancer treatment is additionally complicated during pregnancy. We have to balance timing of treatment for the mother with doing as little harm as possible to the developing fetus. Often these goals are directly contradictory. Surgery for the mother could result in preterm labor or miscarriage of the fetus. Meanwhile, chemotherapy that might be lifesaving for the mother could have significant developmental effects on the fetus. In other words, the successful management of both breast cancer and pregnancy requires an exquisite balance and an expert team that will include your surgeon and oncologist working in partnership with an obstetrician who has expertise in high-risk pregnancies, and even possibly a neonatologist in case of prematurity or early delivery. The good news is that for many women in this rare and difficult situation, with the best team in place the outcome for both mother and baby can be excellent.

Decisions about management for women with breast cancer who

are pregnant depends to some degree on how far along the pregnancy is at diagnosis. Management options are usually broken down by trimester, according to when you were diagnosed. Let's start with the last trimester first, as options for management become more complicated the earlier you are in the course of your pregnancy.

1. **Third trimester.** By the time you are in your third trimester the fetus is of course on its way to enter the world. At thirty-five weeks, the baby and its organ systems are almost fully mature and can be safely delivered early, with some special preparations. So in many cases when breast cancer is diagnosed during the third trimester, the strategy is to delay treatment for just a few weeks, with a plan to induce labor or perform a caesarean section so that the baby can be delivered early. The mother's breast cancer treatment can then begin as soon as possible after delivery without having any effects on the baby.

   In the event that the breast cancer diagnosis is advanced and treatment needs to start immediately, there is a large amount of data showing that surgery *can* be performed safely during pregnancy, with fetal monitoring and an obstetrics team standing by in case of need for delivery. Chemotherapy can also usually be initiated during this phase of pregnancy if needed without a huge amount of risk because the baby's organs are already almost fully formed by now, and this final phase of pregnancy mostly involves final growth and development.

2. **Second trimester.** Women in their middle trimester cannot usually wait to complete the pregnancy to initiate treatment, and unless you are diagnosed during the very earliest part of this trimester, termination of the pregnancy will most likely not be an option for you. During the middle trimester, therefore, we have to focus on optimizing treatment for the mother while doing as little harm as possible to the developing fetus. Surgery— lumpectomy, mastectomy—can certainly be performed safely during pregnancy, but the risks of preterm labor or miscarriage are much higher during this precarious stage of pregnancy. Preterm labor early in the second trimester, when the fetus is only

on the cusp of viability, can lead to significant and severe long-term health and development disorders for the baby. Often surgery can be delayed a few weeks, which can make a big difference for fetal development during this critical period.

With respect to chemotherapy, the growth and development of major organs in the fetus will be in process, and chemotherapy can affect this development. Certain types of chemotherapy have been shown to be safer during pregnancy than others, so a top-notch medical oncologist who is familiar with this data can help you make these critical decisions regarding the best agents for treatment.

3. **First trimester.** Women who are diagnosed with breast cancer during the earliest stage of pregnancy often have the toughest decisions to make. A normal pregnancy lasts the better part of forty weeks, and so treatment clearly cannot wait until pregnancy is completed. Obviously treatment for cancer can increase risk for an unborn child, but the pregnancy itself can increase the risk for the mother too. In the months ahead your body will continually release larger amounts of estrogen and progesterone into your system to support the pregnancy, which may have a dangerous fueling effect on a tumor if you have a hormonally sensitive cancer.

Termination of the pregnancy at this early stage for the benefit and health of the mother and her treatment may be considered. The decision to terminate a pregnancy is heartbreaking under any circumstance and is especially fraught after a breast cancer diagnosis. For many women, a termination would conflict with religious beliefs, or simply derail a long-held dream to become a mother. A woman may feel very differently about a termination if it's her first pregnancy versus a subsequent pregnancy where there are already children in the picture for whom she wants to stay healthy. Although the decision making may seem like a devastating process, with no good options available, with the right guidance and the right support you can get through it. Whatever decision you make should be done with the support of your doctors and those closest to you.

In some situations, it is possible to carry the pregnancy to term if the diagnosis is made late in the first trimester and the tumor is not advanced at the time of detection. If you do decide to take this path, you need to understand that while delaying treatment can have major consequences for *you,* proceeding with treatment can have significant consequences for the fetus and its normal development. In the first trimester of your pregnancy, major organ formation is taking place, and any type of treatment can dramatically affect this critical phase of embryonic and fetal development. Again, there is no one clear-cut road map to managing this extremely difficult situation, and there will be many factors to take into account, both personal and medical.

Pregnancy *after* breast cancer treatment

It's important to know that the main treatments given to improve survival from breast cancer in premenopausal women, chemotherapy and the drug tamoxifen, can affect your fertility and your ability to have children in the future. Certain types of chemotherapy, including those commonly given for breast cancer treatment, can put a woman into menopause, both functionally and symptomatically. The likelihood of going into menopause after chemotherapy is related to your proximity to menopause prior to starting treatment: a forty-year-old is much more likely to go into early menopause than a thirty-year-old.

If you do remain fertile after chemotherapy—or if you did not need chemotherapy in the first place—the other potential obstacle to becoming pregnant in the future is the drug tamoxifen. As we have seen, tamoxifen is an estrogen-receptor blocker that reduces the risk of breast cancer recurrence and is recommended as part of treatment for most premenopausal women with hormone-sensitive tumors. Tamoxifen is a pill, taken once a day, and is usually started after the other components of treatment (surgery, chemotherapy, radiation) have been completed. No woman should get pregnant while on tamoxifen—it's a teratogen, meaning it causes birth defects. Until recently, the standard course of tamoxifen treatment had been five years, but since then, the recommendations changed to extend the course of treatment for many women to ten years (see chapter 9 for more information on tamoxifen). This puts many younger women with a breast cancer diagnosis in a terrible bind. Of course they want to optimize their chances of survival by taking the drug, but if they stay on tamoxifen for ten or even just five years they could effectively eradicate their childbearing window completely. While it is never recommended, some women do start tamoxifen and then consider discontinuing treatment so that they can become pregnant, knowing this may increase their risk of recurrence. This is an extremely difficult choice for a woman who prioritizes both survival and having a family. A good breast oncologist will help guide you through this decision-making process and help you to understand the risks and benefits for you personally. As with every decision regarding breast cancer treatment, one size does not fit all.

Fertility preservation

If you are of childbearing age and you have been diagnosed with breast cancer, your options for fertility preservation should be discussed up front. The sooner you have these discussions after diagnosis, the sooner you will be able to make decisions about your fertility with the least compromise and delay of your cancer care. It's important that you see a fertility specialist *before* surgery to get a sense of your options and plan your care. Equally, seeing your medical oncologist from day one can also be helpful in forming a cohesive plan.

Fertility preservation procedures involve egg harvesting and freezing (usually involving hormonal stimulation to retrieve an increased number of eggs within a cycle), as well as embryo freezing. While there are many medications that are used for ovarian stimulation in treating women with infertility issues, not all of these hormonal stimulants are safe in women with breast cancer, especially when the cancer is hormonally sensitive. Much research has been devoted to identifying hormonal agents and fertility drugs that can be given safely to women with breast cancer without incurring a large increased risk. A fertility specialist who specializes in or has experience in oncofertility (fertility preservation related to cancer) will know which are the most suitable medications to use to induce ovulation in a woman with breast cancer.

If your medical team determines that you are a candidate for fertility preservation, then your treatment and egg harvesting will usually take place in the interval between surgery and chemotherapy. Although many women are good candidates for fertility preservation, a very advanced breast cancer in a woman with borderline fertility may lead a specialist to question the safety of delaying breast cancer treatment to preserve eggs that may not be viable or healthy.

A WORD TO THE WISE

Good preparation and coordination between your specialists will provide you with the most options for fertility with the least amount of delay in your cancer care. If you wait to see the fertility specialist until after surgery is complete, it could take time to get an appointment, then more time to schedule the beginning of fertility treatment. As fertility procedures usually need to be coordinated with your menstrual cycle, this can be a source of further delay, which in turn delays the start date for your chemotherapy. So once again, when it comes to fertility preservation, it's vital to get all your appointments arranged before surgery. Most full-service breast centers will help you with referrals and may even have their own oncofertility program.

Fertility preservation: how it works

Here is how the fertility preservation process is usually sequenced:

1. You see the surgeon to understand and plan timing of surgery.
2. Once your surgery date is planned, you see the fertility specialist and medical oncologist (preferably before surgery), to determine if you are a candidate for fertility preservation.
3. Surgery for breast cancer proceeds.
4. Fertility drugs are given to induce ovulation and facilitate retrieval of multiple eggs. This process usually needs to be timed with your menstrual cycle.

5. The egg harvesting and retrieval procedure is performed.
6. Your medical oncologist is ready and waiting to start chemotherapy as soon as possible based on your previous consultation.

Goserelin

A new study has shown that goserelin—also called Zoladex—is effective in preserving ovarian function during chemotherapy. What happens is that the drug effectively suppresses ovarian function, putting your ovaries to sleep while you are being treated, which in turn protects them during exposure to the chemotherapy. A recent study showed that adding goserelin to chemotherapy in women with breast cancer under the age of fifty reduced the ovarian failure rate due to chemotherapy from 22 percent to 8 percent. On follow-up, more women in the group that received goserelin ultimately had babies successfully than those who did not receive goserelin. It should be noted that only women with non-hormone-sensitive breast cancers (estrogen/progesterone negative) were included in this study (see chapter 8 for more information on hormonally sensitive cancers), so this new option for improved fertility preservation can be considered in many but not all cases.

Finances and fertility preservation

While insurance does cover most aspects of breast cancer care—including surgery, chemotherapy, reconstruction, and even removal of a healthy other breast—coverage for fertility preservation has never been as universal or robust. With very few exceptions, commercial insurance plans generally do not provide coverage for this service. Meanwhile, the treatments and procedures for fertility preservation are prohibitively expensive: each cycle of egg stimulation and retrieval can cost tens of thousands of dollars, putting this option out of reach even for women who consider themselves financially comfortable. There are some charity organizations that can offer resources to women unable to afford these procedures and help patients identify health care providers who are amenable to performing these services at reduced rates. For more on this, see the online resources section at the end of the book.

Pregnancy *after* breast cancer treatment: when is it safe? And is it safe?

Many women newly diagnosed with breast cancer who are hoping to become pregnant in the future have the same question: "Once I finish my treatment for breast cancer, when is it safe to start trying to get pregnant?" The answer is that there is no standard answer, because it is truly different for each woman. There is no specific, set amount of time after which we *know* pregnancy is safe, just like there is no set amount of time after which we *know* breast cancer can't recur. The goal is always to optimize treatment and its length, and to allow enough time to pass so that you can be reasonably comfortable that based on your tumor type, stage, and treatment, the cancer has a low risk of recurrence (understanding that there are no guarantees). As the timing is determined case by case, it's important to discuss this with your medical team and family to determine the optimal time for *you*.

The other question that comes up with women who want to get pregnant after a breast cancer diagnosis is this one: "Can being pregnant increase the risk of the cancer coming back?" While there had been some suggestion that the high hormone levels of pregnancy could increase the risk of cancer recurrence, most studies indicate that becoming pregnant *after* a diagnosis of breast cancer does not decrease likelihood of survival, as long as the woman is otherwise healthy and has recovered from her breast cancer.

Breastfeeding after breast cancer treatment

If you had a mastectomy, your breast no longer functions to produce milk, and breastfeeding from that side is not an option. It's also important to be aware that you may not be able to breastfeed with a preserved breast even if you have a lumpectomy, due to scarring effects from both the surgery and the radiation. If the other healthy breast was not removed, then breastfeeding from this breast can be successful.

THE TAKEAWAY

- Breast cancer during pregnancy is complicated but not impossible. Make sure you have the best team.
- Treatment options vary and are impacted by the trimester of diagnosis. Balancing the best treatment for you with the safety of the baby is critical.
- Pregnancy after breast cancer is also complicated but not impossible. Again, balancing your own optimal treatment with the timing of future pregnancy is critical.

CHAPTER 18

Recurrence

devastation and finding hope

y patient Janice was fifty-seven when she first came to see me. She had a small, aggressive breast cancer that had spread to a few lymph nodes under her arm, but after surgery and chemotherapy, she made a swift recovery. Three years after her surgery, however, Janice developed some pain in her upper back. Initially, she tried to ignore it, thinking it was related to straining while lifting a heavy box. But the pain persisted, and she called her oncologist for advice. Her oncologist ordered a bone scan, which showed some small spots on Janice's spine and one on her right hip. When we compared these spots to the bone scan she'd had immediately before her surgery, they were new and therefore suspicious. A needle biopsy was done. The breast cancer had spread to the bone.

Janice came back to my office, understandably distraught. How could this have happened three years after surgery? Wasn't she supposed to be cured? I explained that it is our sincerest hope that every single patient will be cured, but that there is always a possibility that cancer will come back. As much as any of us like to think otherwise, where cancer is concerned, there are factors that are beyond our control.

For most people, the risk of cancer coming back after a breast cancer diagnosis is fairly low. If you're diagnosed with DCIS, or noninvasive cancer, the odds of the cancer coming back could be as low as 1 to 2 percent. For patients where the cancer was very aggressive the first time around—as was the case with Janice—there is a much higher risk of cancer returning, sometimes as high as 50 percent. Although we can never predict which patients will be affected and which will remain cancer free, what we do know is that if breast cancer is going to come back, it will most likely recur within the first two to three years after treatment. For some it can occur much later, even ten to fifteen years after the original diagnosis. When cancer does recur, it can take many courses. Some women with recurrence can live for many years taking medication that keeps the cancer at bay. Some women have a more rapidly declining course, where none of the many medications and treatments we have to offer seem to work. And while there is always room for optimism, there is no doubt that anytime cancer returns this is a devastating scenario for patients and their families (and the doctors who take care of them, as well).

For Janice it was extremely demoralizing to find herself in the situation of having to face treatment all over again, as well as the realization that this time the cancer was no longer curable. She was about to become a grandmother, and she was helping her daughter plan for the baby shower and birth. She was simply too busy for cancer, and she felt fine! I reassured Janice that there were still many options for her treatment, most of which would allow her to do all the things she still needed and wanted to do.

As I explain to my patients, there are good reasons to remain optimistic, even after cancer comes back. Newer, better treatments are becoming available all the time. And for women who were treated a long time ago, the options for treatment may have changed and improved significantly since the first time they were treated.

When it comes to recurrence, it's important to know there are two types: local and systemic.

LOCAL RECURRENCE

Local recurrence is when a woman who underwent lumpectomy the first time around has the cancer return in the same breast. The likelihood of local recurrence after lumpectomy and radiation is low (approximately 5 percent), but it can happen. Some of the signs of recurrence in the breast include

1. A new finding on your yearly mammogram or other imaging test
2. A new lump that you feel in the breast, near the previous scar or elsewhere
3. Changes to the breast skin or nipple, such as redness, thickening, pulling, or indentation
4. New nipple discharge

Treatment of local recurrence after previous lumpectomy

Mastectomy

Recurrence in the same breast is treatable and potentially curable again.

However, mastectomy is the recommended procedure the second time around (lumpectomy and radiation go together, and radiation is no longer an option, as it cannot be given to the same area twice). Reconstruction with mastectomy can be more complicated in the setting of recurrence, since radiation changes affect the skin in a way that makes the skin less elastic (see chapter 7, on reconstruction, and chapter 10, on radiation side effects), but it can be done in most cases, and may certainly cushion the blow of needing a mastectomy.

Treatment of local recurrence after previous mastectomy

Local recurrence can also happen after a mastectomy, although with little breast tissue left, the likelihood is very low. Some of the signs of recurrence after mastectomy include

1. A lump or raised bump in or under the skin, especially near the previous mastectomy scar
2. Changes to the skin, including redness or thickening

Treatment of local recurrence after mastectomy can involve a variety of different approaches, including surgery to remove the recurrence if it is confined to a limited area. Other options for treatment include radiation, chemotherapy, and endocrine therapy, or a combination of these.

Lymph nodes

If you have a local recurrence and only had a few lymph nodes checked the first time as part of a sentinel node biopsy procedure, then in some situations it will be recommended to undergo a repeat sentinel node biopsy procedure to check for spread to remaining nodes. If you had all of your nodes removed during prior surgery, there are usually no nodes left to check, and nothing further in the nodes is recommended as part of the second surgical procedure.

Regional recurrence

Regional recurrence usually refers to cancer that has recurred in the region of the breast, usually the lymph nodes under your arm or in the neck. In many cases treatment for regional recurrence, like local recurrence, can involve surgically removing the area of recurrence, but also can involve radiation, chemotherapy, hormonal therapy, or some combination thereof.

Chemotherapy and endocrine therapy

With local recurrence, after surgery, your doctors will determine your need for additional treatment—including chemotherapy, endocrine therapy, or both—on a case-by-case basis. In some cases, such as recurrence of DCIS alone, no additional treatment may be needed once mastectomy is done. There are some chemotherapeutic treatments that can only be given once, so if you have a local recurrence and need chemotherapy again, different options may be considered. For patients who were on a specific hormonal treatment prior to the recurrence, such as tamoxifen, usually that particular medicine is stopped, as obviously the tamoxifen, which was being given to *prevent* recurrence, hasn't been working. But there are usually other options to turn to, such as removal of the ovaries or suppression of ovarian function with medication to prevent further estrogen production, with aromatase inhibitors to follow.

Radiation therapy

Radiation can also be part of treatment for local or regional recurrence, mainly when the area had not been radiated previously, since radiation can be given only once to each particular area of the body.

SYSTEMIC RECURRENCE

Systemic recurrence, or metastasis (meaning that the cancer has spread through your system or body), is much more serious than local recurrence and is synonymous with stage 4 disease. For breast cancer patients, the most common areas of spread are the bone, liver, lungs and brain. Tragically, stage 4 disease cannot be cured.

Many times a patient will say, "Well, if there is just one spot in my liver, why can't you just remove that spot, like you did with the lumpectomy in my breast?" The problem is that when the cancer has spread to other parts of the body, it's no longer helpful to remove the new site of the disease, since there will still be remaining cells circulating in the body that will quickly reappear elsewhere.

My message to patients in this situation is that there is still reason for hope. There are usually many options for medical treatment, and it is possible for patients to develop a durable response to treatment, enabling them to live with the cancer under control for a number of years. For the vast majority of women, however, the cancer will keep returning in some way, since circulating cells can never be completely eradicated and metastatic cancer can develop resistance to effective treatment. New treatments are being developed all the time, which means that some women can remain in longer periods of remission by repeatedly switching to an alternative treatment after they become resistant to the prior one. The more options for treatment, the more potential that patients will be able to survive for longer periods of time. I've seen patients who have lived ten years or more after developing stage 4 disease, but not enough fare this well.

For women with metastatic disease, there are many paths for treatment. Treatment usually depends on the extent and location of the recurrence, the profile of the cancer, what was previously used for treatment, and many other factors. What's critical is that you find a specialized breast medical oncologist who is aware of all the existing treatment agents available, any clinical trials that might be appropriate, and new treatments that are coming down the pipeline. If you weren't already at a specialized center for your first treatment, you should definitely explore this option now, and at least get a second opinion regarding what additional options may be available at a major cancer center. (For more on clinical trials, see the section of online resources.)

Symptoms of recurrence

For most patients when the cancer comes back, it is usually detected by symptoms specific to the organ system involved. For example, recurrence in the bone can lead to new pain in that particular area. Other potential symptoms include abdominal pain or weight loss, jaundice (appearing yellow), new headaches, seizures, changes in vision, persistent cough, or shortness of breath.

How recurrence happens

Many people cannot understand how a person can be "cured" one day and be diagnosed with recurrent cancer the next. If surgery got most or all of the cancer out and chemotherapy and radiation were supposed to have mopped up the rest, how can recurrence even happen? Here's how.

In most cases, even the smallest breast cancer detected had been growing for some time before it was caught. During this period of growth, the cancer cells multiplied and divided over and over again, and some cancer cells splintered off from the main tumor and escaped into the surrounding blood and lymphatic vessels. Cells that spread to lymph nodes can certainly be trapped in those lymph nodes and removed at the time of surgery, but cells can also go beyond the lymph nodes, traveling via lymphatics into the circulatory system. Even early-stage cancers that originally had no lymph node involvement can recur and develop metastatic disease. While it's not common, cancer cells can bypass lymphatics and lymph nodes and travel via surrounding blood vessels. Cancer cells can continue to circulate and go anywhere the blood vessels will take them, or they can home in on other organs in the body, where they take up residence and continue to grow and divide in that one particular spot.

Why weren't these escaping cells identified the first time the cancer was treated? Although scans of the body can detect if there is *obvious* spread to these other organs, for women with early stage breast cancer there rarely is anything that shows up on a scan. There is a limit to what scans can tell us: they won't show extremely tiny spots of cancer, and they definitely can't show us if there are individual cells circulating in the body. Neither will any blood test, or any other test for that matter. So the first time around we perform our surgery and give our treatments—chemotherapy, hormonal therapy, radiation—with the hope that if microscopic spread has already taken place, the treatments will scavenge those cells and kill them before they take up residence someplace in the body.

Here's the problem: these treatments don't work 100 percent of the time. So *if* cells have spread, and *if* the treatments we give don't affect them, the cancer cells can persist and take hold someplace, developing into metastases, or spread. This is why and how recurrence happens.

MYTH: "I should be getting frequent scans and blood tests so that if I do develop metastasis, it will be detected early."

Given the ominous nature of stage 4 disease, the next obvious question is, why don't we scan for spread regularly after a first diagnosis, so that we can detect it early if it does return? The reason we don't scan or test for metastasis is that there really is no "early" stage 4 disease, and thus no real opportunity to intervene earlier and increase the chance of cure. It's also important to know that with recurrence, one does not progress from one stage to the next: a woman who was originally diagnosed with stage 1 breast cancer does not recur as stage 2, because once cells have taken up residence elsewhere, she is immediately considered to have stage 4 disease. And with stage 4 disease, either you respond well to treatment and the disease regresses, or you don't and it doesn't. Studies have shown that getting frequent scans after a first cancer diagnosis does not lead to improved survival, which is why we don't scan for stage 4—even if we wish we could.

Biopsies

When there are signs of recurrence, a biopsy of the new site of disease needs to be performed to verify the findings. We also need to find out what is making the tumor grow so it can be treated more effectively. Most metastatic sites mirror the original cancer profile and are the same in terms of estrogen receptor, progesterone receptor, and Her2/neu-positivity (for more on these tumor profiles, see chapter 8). But in approximately 10 to 20 percent of cases, the tumor mutates into something else, and it is critically important to know the new status so that the metastatic lesions can be effectively treated. For example, what if the original tumor was estrogen receptor positive and the new metastatic lesion is estrogen receptor negative? We would know not to waste time trying to treat this more serious disease with a hormonal agent, since it won't work. Even for metastases that do replicate the original tumor, for the majority of patients treatment will be very different the second time around.

THE TAKEAWAY

- With recurrence, remain optimistic if you can.
- Go to a specialized center to make sure you know about the best options that might be available for your particular case.
- Treatment for stage 4 disease can have a variable course, and you may have to switch treatments in order to have a more durable response. More than in any other situation, one size does not fit all.

CHAPTER 19

The 10 Percent

when all else fails

Each year, approximately 300,000 women will be diagnosed with breast cancer in the United States. And survival rates *overall* currently approach 90 percent. This means that of 300,000 women diagnosed this year, approximately 270,000 will be alive in five years or more. It also means that, tragically, 30,000 will not survive. Such a high rate of survival is a reason for optimism, and certainly represents a significant amount of progress since the 1970s, when overall survival was closer to 70 percent. After all, the death rate from breast cancer dropped almost 2 percent per year in the ten years between 2000 and 2010. But the fact remains that while a 10 percent risk of dying may not sound like a high percentage, it represents an incomprehensible number of lives lost.

A small number of women, approximately 5 percent, will have stage 4 disease (incurable cancer) at the time of their original diagnosis with breast cancer. This can represent women who did not get screened or do not have access to care and thus did not have the opportunity for early diagnosis and a better chance for cure.* An interesting and sober-

---

* Webb ML, Cady B, Michaelson JS, et al. A failure analysis of invasive breast cancer: most deaths from disease occur in women not regularly screened. *Cancer*, 2014.

ing study out of Massachusetts showed that of a sample group of women who ultimately died of breast cancer, 71 percent had either *never* had a mammogram (65 percent), or had not gotten one within the previous two years (6 percent). However, the study also included women who, despite being very conscientious and taking every precaution, including yearly mammograms, developed such biologically aggressive disease that it defied early detection. So besides those who are diagnosed at the outset with stage 4 disease, there is no way of knowing or predicting who of those originally treated for cure will later develop stage 4 disease.

While stage 4 disease cannot be cured, it can be treated, even for years. When I work with patients with stage 4 cancer, we often discuss maintaining optimism in this situation. New treatments are being developed all the time that can extend quantity and quality of life. And participating in clinical trials of new drugs can also be a way to receive these promising medications. Patients who have the resources and money may be inclined to spend a significant amount of time traveling around the country searching for experimental trials that could extend both quantity and quality of life. However, it's important to know that when standard treatment options are exhausted, it is mostly purely a matter of chance whether a patient can find a new treatment that offers any level of response and improvement. If you are already receiving care in a major center, then your doctors will be able to tell you about promising trials being done at other institutions and advise if one of these would be right for you.

Even so, there are situations in which we reach a point, as happens with all types of cancer, where it becomes clear that in a particular case we are going to lose the battle. This is one of the most agonizing and heart-wrenching realizations for a woman and her family to have. And for a doctor, there is nothing worse than to give this news and have this discussion. These situations are associated with profound sadness. It is important that patients and their families feel continued connection with their doctors during this time, that they know they are not being abandoned, and that they feel that their needs are being met and all their questions are answered.

Maintaining contact with your physicians

As a surgeon who usually takes care of women in the earliest stages of cancer diagnosis and treatment, I am by no means an expert in the final phases of care. It is usually my medical oncology colleagues who are most deeply involved in the care of women with stage 4 disease, and responsible for providing guidance to our mutual patients during this phase. While there is a misconception that doctors are only focused on the patients we can help or cure, for many of us there is a sincere, heartfelt connection with patients whom we have come to know and care about deeply. I have an ongoing relationship with most women I have taken care of, and often get to know my patients and their families well. The caring and connection do not end when we have nothing more to offer from a medical standpoint. When we reach a point where all treatment options have been exhausted, I know exactly what's at stake. Each woman is the center of a small universe that will be completely shattered after she is gone. Our only goal as physicians is caring for and protecting our patients, and getting to the point where there is nothing left to offer and no way to help represents total failure and utter despair for us as well. There is no consolation for these losses, and my only comfort in these situations is to focus on the role that I was honored to play in my patient's life. And for doctors and scientists, each death drives us harder to find more and better options for the future.

An entire book could be devoted to dealing with the reality of stage 4 breast cancer and its last phases. The course can be a windy road or a steady or precipitous decline. There is no map to take you through this part of the journey, when the options for treatment become fewer and fewer and the end becomes inevitable.

The fight-till-the-end approach versus the comfort-and-care approach: not mutually exclusive

When the doctors who are treating you, usually medical oncologists, indicate that there is nothing else to offer and the cancer is advancing despite all best efforts, most patients and their families retrench and reevaluate. One option is to go elsewhere, as there may be other options out there that might work for you, and there is nothing wrong with looking for those options. Most major cancer centers now list clinical trials for metastatic breast cancer on their websites, and many places may offer some interesting clinical trials for patients who have not had good results from other treatments. Traveling to get other opinions is always an option if a woman is healthy enough. Many women and their families feel that it is important to know that they fought until the end.

But remember, this is also a time when patients and their families are particularly vulnerable to predatory treatments offering false hope. I have seen patients spend thousands of dollars in the last months of life on unapproved and uninvestigated treatments with no potential benefit, just because nothing else has worked. While it may be tempting to explore alternatives when traditional medicine has failed, my advice would be to stick with recognized clinical trials within major medical centers. Try not to exhaust energy, any remaining time there is, or family savings on treatments promoted by snake oil salesmen and their websites. And remember, every treatment has some kind of side effect that can potentially affect quality of life, comfort, and ability to spend meaningful time together in the time that is left.

When it becomes clear that most of the realistic options for treatment and results have been exhausted, another approach is to focus on quality of life and comfort. What are the remaining things that need to be said and done? How can you maximize your time with those who are closest? It is critically important to know that this approach in *no way* constitutes "giving up." Dignity, comfort, and choosing one's own destiny in the final stages are all equally heroic.

Focusing on what you, the patient, want

For patients and their families, the end of life is associated with the most complicated range of emotions imaginable. Feelings can range over the course of hours from shock to numbness, from grief to rage, from fear to courage, from despair to acceptance. It is always important to keep in the forefront of your mind that there is no one right path, and that as the patient, you are the only person who should be dictating the course of events. Family pressures to "try something new" and "not give up" are common, especially from those who have not seen the full extent of what you have endured. You are the only one who should make the decision about what measures should be taken and when.

This is also a time to focus on the support you and your family need at this critical juncture. Support can come in many different forms: counseling, being with family and friends, support groups, and even medication. This is the time to prioritize yourself and put your needs first without any apologies. Reaching for support is a sign of strength, not weakness, and can improve the quality of how you live. Reaching out to your doctors during this time and having your doctors come visit you either in the hospital or at home may also be an important part of your continued care.

End-of-life care

Palliative care

At some point, when the cancer is advancing despite everyone's best efforts, palliative care may be appropriate. Palliative care addresses issues related to pain management and symptom control. Metastatic breast cancer frequently involves the bones, and so pain control is critical. Lung involvement can make breathing difficult—palliative procedures can take fluid off the lung and prevent it from reaccumulating. Palliative care and treatment are not mutually exclusive, and pursuing palliative care does *not* necessarily mean giving up on treatment options. The two processes, treatment and palliative care, can be complementary, and most major medical centers have well-developed palliative care programs where common goals for you and your family can be addressed by a coordinated team of specialists. Palliative care programs and services can be both inpatient and outpatient.

But palliative care can also often mean transitioning a woman out of active treatment mode and into comfort care mode, where the focus is on ensuring she is at ease and that her pain is minimized. Often these care measures can be given at home in a more comfortable setting surrounded by family and friends.

Hospice

Hospice care comes into play when death is imminent and the focus shifts entirely to comfort and pain control. Hospice services can be delivered in a hospital or care facility or at home, and can involve everything from pain management to assisting with basic activities such as eating and trips to the bathroom. Equally as important, hospice caregivers can help provide psychological, social, and spiritual support during this time. Hospice care usually is initiated in the final months to weeks of life.

Hospice is also for friends and family

Hospice care can be an important part of supporting the people who have been providing loving care for you all along during this incredibly difficult time. When you have hospice caregivers available to tend to many of your physical needs, your loved ones can focus less on *doing for you* and more on *being with you*. These are the times to express gratitude, love, and that you will always be with them in spirit. Perhaps there will be opportunities for you to address any unresolved issues, which can bring profound peace to both you and your family members, and to have a say in how you will be remembered.

CHAPTER 20

The Future

moving forward with hope and optimism

After surgery is completed, I usually see my patients in my office one week afterward to check on wound healing and to discuss results from surgery, then three months later to make sure they are continuing to heal well and have completed the additional recommended treatments. After that, we continue with routine follow-up visits twice a year for two to three years, and then yearly after that. What I've seen is that life after breast cancer can be more complicated than many people expect. For a period of time, it can feel like you are waiting for the other shoe to drop. Will the cancer come back? If so, will it be in the same breast? In the other breast? Somewhere else?

What I've also seen is that as time passes, the immediate fear of cancer does eventually begin to fade into the background. For some women it takes longer than for others. I have had patients who can go through most of the year without even thinking about cancer until they know their appointment for their yearly mammogram is approaching, at which point they can't rest until they hear me say, "Your mammogram and exam are normal. See you in a year!" For others, thoughts of cancer are much more frequent, and they have to work through their anxiety so that daily life can go on.

Whether you fall into the former or latter group, you should know that your fears and concerns are completely normal, and part of a very human reaction to an extremely stressful experience. If you are struggling to keep your anxiety under control, however, you may decide to seek counseling. Many cancer survivors also find great consolation in support groups—talking with others who have been there can help remind you that you're not alone.

As I always tell my patients, life after cancer treatment means learning to accept the limits of what you—or your doctors—can control. All of us who are cancer doctors would love to tell each and every patient, "You're cured forever. The cancer is never coming back." But that's not something that any cancer doctor can honestly guarantee. There's always a small chance of recurrence. It's simply the reality of cancer. Instead, we have to work with what we can control and try to accept that which is beyond our control. Thankfully, for most women, if we do the best we can with treatment and the things we can control, it's usually enough.

What you *can't* control after treatment

1. **Tumor biology.** There are many factors that can help us predict risk of recurrence. Tumor size and lymph node status help us stage cancer and are important pieces of information for determining treatment. They also tell us much about tumor biology and likely outcome. There are even tests now, such as the Oncotype DX (see chapter 9), that can tell us about the biologic behavior and aggressiveness of your cancer and its likelihood of recurrence. But these numbers and predictors are overall percentages. And overall the survival rate for newly diagnosed breast cancer approaches 90 percent, which is better than ever. What these numbers can't predict with absolute certainty, however, is your *individual* outcome. For any given woman, there is no way of knowing or foreseeing the future. But this also applies to so many factors beyond breast cancer! Your doctors can be a good source of reassurance, but once treatment is completed, then the rest of life and how things will play out remains to be seen. And again, this is not just for breast cancer.

2. **Recurrence.** With good treatment, the likelihood of local recurrence after both lumpectomy and mastectomy is low. After lumpectomy, careful surveillance gives us the best chance of early detection again in the unlikely scenario that the cancer does recur. Systemic recurrence, on the other hand, is not something that can be detected "early." Once the best treatment for the initial cancer has been given, the risk of systemic recurrence cannot be definitively determined for any individual. Again, for most women the likelihood of recurrence like this is low, but it is never zero. In this sense, eradicating any potential risk of recurrence simply isn't possible.

What you *can* control after treatment

1. **A regular screening schedule recommended by your doctor.** Regular follow-up visits to your doctor as recommended by him or her are an important part of your care. For women who have had a lumpectomy, a regular screening schedule means that if there is a new finding in the breast, either on examination or on imaging, it can potentially be caught early and treated for cure again. Even with mastectomy, examination of the chest wall and remaining lymph nodes under the arm are important parts of follow-up care. Doctors who are at the forefront of the field will also update you if exciting new options for treatment become available. As an example, the recent extension of tamoxifen from five years to ten was an update that for appropriate patients further reduces their risk of recurrence. For many of my patients who were about to complete their planned five years of tamoxifen, further discussion with me and their oncologist led to a change in plan to continue for another five, thereby potentially further reducing their risk of recurrence. In other words, ongoing conversations with your doctors are important for continued well-being.

2. **Overall physical health.** Speaking of continued well-being, as your breast cancer diagnosis and treatment move further and fur-

ther into the past, you may find that you want to reevaluate and reassess various lifestyle factors. Are there any lifestyle factors where you may have room for improvement? Some, like alcohol intake and weight, affect both overall well-being *and* breast cancer recurrence risk (see chapter 13 for more on this). Others, like smoking, affect overall health, and in a very significant way—so much so that for women who smoke, the risk of breast cancer recurrence might actually be a less significant health concern moving forward than their risk for developing lung cancer, emphysema, cardiovascular disease, and other potentially fatal smoking-related complications. Some of my patients newly diagnosed with breast cancer reveal that it has been years since they have been to see a gynecologist for a Pap smear or general checkup. And for these women, a resolution to get back on track with a more conscientious approach to regular health maintenance and prevention is one potential positive outcome. In the months to first few years after treatment, getting back to normal is always a priority, but for some it's a new normal, and for some it can be a better normal. When you are ready, use your doctors, oncologists, or general practitioners for advice and guidance to find out how you can improve your overall health.

3. **Overall emotional health.** Quality of life is just as important as quantity of life. So an important part of moving forward is making sure that you are on track to deriving enjoyment and pleasure out of every day—at least as much as you had before your diagnosis, if not more. A certain amount of stress and fear is an extremely normal part of being diagnosed with breast cancer, while undergoing all aspects of treatment, and during the aftermath as well. But if extreme anxiety or distress regarding recurrence becomes an ongoing struggle or obstacle to happiness or emotional health, it may be time to seek counseling or other methods of support. If you are cured of breast cancer but cannot enjoy life, what has really been accomplished?

Moving forward with optimism—and leaving breast cancer in the background

I can't imagine a more fulfilling, honorable profession than treating and helping to cure women with breast cancer. For me and my team, it is an everyday occurrence. And yet every day is a remarkable gift, uniquely satisfying, and about as far from "routine" as one can get. And with every day come new opportunities: to make someone feel better, to give someone hope, to save a life. While those of us taking care of women with breast cancer are privileged to play an incredibly central role in our patients' lives for a short period of time while they are undergoing active treatment, our ultimate goal is to fade into the background. As time passes, frequent consultations and discussions regarding surgery turn into less frequent follow-up visits every few months. Eventually these follow-up visits become yearly. And in time, my yearly visits with patients become less focused on talking about cancer and more about catching up on their lives.

When I first met one of my patients, Muriel, twelve years ago, she just wanted to recover from her breast cancer surgery so that she could see the birth of her first grandchild. That grandchild is now about to have her bat mitzvah, so we spent most of her yearly checkup visit gossiping about the dress Muriel plans on wearing. Another patient, Helen, a young woman with no family history of breast cancer, was diagnosed with breast cancer at age thirty-four while pregnant with her first child. At the time Helen couldn't imagine being at her son's fifth birthday, but there she was in my office five years later (and pregnant again, no less!), scrolling through the pictures of her son's birthday party on her phone.

The goal of every patient and doctor is to find a path forward, leaving breast cancer in the background. And with the right treatment, this goal is truly realistic for most women who are newly diagnosed. Imagine the stories you will tell five and ten years from now. These are the stories that keep everyone going forward. Including me.

Acknowledgments

The idea for this book was born out of a conversation I had with my dear friend Beth Kobliner Shaw, who herself happens to be a best-selling writer. I still vividly remember the phone conversation as she made the case for me to write a book to reach even more women than the ones I actually took care of myself. I listened to what she had to say and bounced ideas off of her, and my inner wheels started spinning as I started to wind the coiled office phone cord tightly around my finger. She subsequently provided immense support in too many ways to count, including giving me the "gift" of an editor to work with early on to get me started. I can safely say that my friendship with her was directly responsible for launching me into writing this book.

Paul Podlucky, another dear friend and the most brilliant hair colorist and stylist (yes, proud to say that I see him regularly), was the next person along the way who was instrumental in getting this project completed. He connected me to Luke Janklow and the incredible Emma Parry at the Janklow Agency. Emma, you are a godsend. You connected me to Eve Claxton, our third E-migo, a brilliant editor who worked with me on the manuscript. Eve, we clicked immediately. Your editorial and organizational talent helped me deliver a book I am so proud of. You both came to the Center, you saw the potential and value of writing this book, and you truly made it happen. Emma, I will always be so appreciative of your efforts and your amazing work to get the book to where it needed to be . . . in the hands of Marnie Cochran.

Marnie, with your insights and expertise, I knew this book was in the best of hands, and you made this book the best it could possibly be. It has been a true joy working with you and getting to know you, and I am beyond appreciative that you made this book a reality. A big thank-you also to Nancy Delia, Cindy Murray, Allison Schuster, and Nicole Morano from Random House and the rest of the Random House publishing staff: I know that getting a book published required a team and to give this book a life, I had the most phenomenal team.

In some ways, this team is similar to the people I work with in my "day job" at the Dubin Breast Center and at Mount Sinai Hospital: a team with no weak links. Melissa Bellino, we have been on an amazing journey together to build the Dubin Breast Center and make it what it has become in a very short period of time: a leading breast center. Your intelligence, skill, competence, and spunk are really beyond compare. Lynn MacDougall, my loyal and wonderful nurse, we have worked together for years to deliver the highest level of care to our patients. I am so proud and lucky to work with you. And the same for Raina Caridi, Deborah Orringer, Melanie Santiago, and Trissa Williams. In addition to the wonderful care you deliver to our patients, you make it fun to come to work every day.

Heartfelt thanks to Eva and Glenn Dubin, my partners in the Dubin Center. We launched our joint vision of optimal breast cancer care, and this further compelled me to deliver the written version of what we do every day in the Center. Thank you for your support, your generosity, and your incredible friendship. And Eva, as a partner you have shown me that it's possible to make such a dream into reality *and* have so much fun along the way.

Thank you to the leadership at Mount Sinai Hospital and Health System: Dr. Dennis Charney, Dr. Ken Davis, and Jeff Silberstein, who, along with the Dubins, recruited me to Mount Sinai and were instrumental in giving me the opportunity of a lifetime to develop a Center and deliver care in breast cancer at the highest level.

Thanks to my parents, Loni and Jeff Rush, who have been so supportive to me and our family in every way and all along the way. You are a huge part of all of my successes.

Time is a zero-sum game. The more time you spend on work, the less time there is to do other things. Like many working moms I struggle every day with trying to get it all done, and it's usually the kids and the husband who get the short end of the stick, more so when you take on an "extra" job or project like writing a book. One day my daughter, Lolo, was trying to get my attention, while I was intent on finishing a paragraph I was writing, and I didn't even look up. She kept on talking and talking, and finally, seeing that I was only half or not-at-all listening, she said, "You know, Mom, *The Optimist's Guide to Breast Cancer* (the working title for the book at that time) is turning into *The Pessimist's Guide to Lolo Time.* I got the message and stepped away from the computer screen. But there were many other occasions when book time cut into family time, and I am just so grateful to Lauren and Zack, my two kids, for their understanding, and their love.

I am so grateful to my amazing husband, Jeffrey. Honey, you have always been there for me, and you have always pushed me to go beyond my comfort zone. And your devotion to our family, your own patients, and your companies truly make the world a better place. I adore you and love you.

Lastly, to all of my patients who I have had the honor and privilege to care for: I have learned something from each and every one of you, and each one of you, in some way, inspired me to write this book.

Appendix 1

some of the most common breast cancer myths—

and the truth

Rumors, misinformation, and half-truths: breast cancer seems to attract more of these than almost any other disease. By the time a new patient has come to see me for the first time, she's usually learned all kinds of "facts" about breast cancer from friends, from family members, and from looking online—and is terrified about her prospects as a result. Although I'm not entirely sure why this should be the case, I think it has to do with how common the disease is. Everyone seems to know something about it and is willing to share their information, some of which is true, but most of which isn't applicable to any *individual* case. Breast cancer is also predominantly a women's disease, and I suspect that in general, women tend to share more, which can cut both ways. What I do know is that breast cancer myths generate a huge amount of anxiety for patients. When a new patient comes to my office, what she's looking for is clarity and a trusted source of information, so that she can make informed decisions about her treatment and recovery without any more stress and anxiety than necessary.

Over my many years of treating breast cancer patients, I've heard every myth in the book (or on the web). Here are a few of the biggest and most commonly mentioned misconceptions out there. Most of them have been brought up in previous chapters, but all are worth repeating.

MYTH: "Needle biopsies spread cancer."

TRUTH: Needle biopsies are a critical tool for diagnosing breast cancer and do not spread breast cancer.

MYTH: "Mammograms cause cancer."

TRUTH: Mammograms are associated with one of the lowest doses of radiation exposure of all radiology tests. Even when multiple pictures are taken—which happens when we perform a biopsy—the overall exposure is low, and is *not* associated with increased risk of cancer.

MYTH: "If you don't have a history of breast cancer in your family, you don't need to start mammograms until you're older."

TRUTH: Having your first mammogram at age forty is the recommendation for breast cancer screening for the general population with no specific breast cancer risk factors.

MYTH: "Cancer grows and spreads quickly; time is of the essence."

TRUTH: Breast cancer usually grows over the course of months and even, in some cases, years. While it's never a good idea to delay diagnosing and treating breast cancer for any considerable length of time, days or even weeks will not make a difference in the potential for cure.

MYTH: "If you have no family history of breast cancer, you really aren't at much risk."

TRUTH: It's important to know that 80 to 90 percent of women newly diagnosed with breast cancer have no family history of breast cancer. In other words, we are all at risk, whether there is a family history or not.

MYTH: "If you have a family history of breast cancer, you will definitely get breast cancer."

TRUTH: While it's true that having a family history of breast cancer raises your risk to above that of the general population, it does not necessarily mean you will get breast cancer in the future.

MYTH: "Mammograms don't really do anything to reduce risk of death from breast cancer."

TRUTH: The mammogram is the *only* test that has been shown to reduce the risk of dying from breast cancer by detecting cancer earlier, thereby increasing the chance for cure.

MYTH: "Mammograms are a fail-safe to prevent breast cancer."

TRUTH: Wrong on two counts. First, approximately 10 to 15 percent of breast cancers won't show up on mammograms at all and are therefore missed by routine mammography. Second, mammograms don't *prevent* breast cancer; they detect it. But they can reduce the risk of dying from breast cancer by detecting it early.

MYTH: "If you have a lump and the mammogram is normal, you have nothing to worry about."

TRUTH: Approximately 10 to 15 percent of breast cancers cannot be seen on mammogram. Therefore, a normal mammogram can't guarantee that you don't have breast cancer. A new or suspicious lump should always prompt further investigation, even when a mammogram is normal.

MYTH: "If you have a lump in your breast, it's definitely breast cancer."

TRUTH: There are normal causes of new breast lumps besides breast cancer. These include cysts, benign breast tissue, and even benign tumors. These can be differentiated from cancer by imaging, examination, and biopsy if necessary.

MYTH: "Breast cancer always comes in the form of a lump."

TRUTH: The smallest breast cancers detected may not be big enough to form a lump that you or your doctor can feel. Approximately 20 to 25 percent of all new breast cancers detected are DCIS (stage 0 breast cancer), which commonly shows up as microcalcifications on a mammogram but which cannot be felt.

MYTH: "Breast implants increase your risk of breast cancer."

TRUTH: Not true. Breast implants do not increase one's risk of developing breast cancer.

MYTH: "Women with larger breasts have a greater chance of getting breast cancer."

TRUTH: Not true. Breast size does not factor into one's risk of getting breast cancer.

MYTH: "You can treat your cancer by altering the pH of your diet."

TRUTH: The pH of the body cannot be altered at will or by dietary or lifestyle changes, although various states of severe illness can. Therefore, the course or treatment of breast cancer cannot be altered in any way by trying to change physiologic pH.

MYTH: "You can starve your cancer by eating less sugar."

TRUTH: Dietary sugar consumption does not directly fuel breast cancer cell growth. Everything we eat gets converted, at the cellular level, to sugar, and this is necessary to feed cells, both good and bad. While it's true you can improve your health by eating less sugary foods—they are usually associated with low nutritional value and obesity, which can increase one's risk of breast cancer—you can't "starve" your cancer by eating less sugar.

MYTH: "Underwire bras can cause cancer."

TRUTH: Not true.

MYTH: "Using deodorant or antiperspirant can cause breast cancer."

TRUTH: Not true (thankfully).

MYTH: "Caffeine can cause breast cancer."

TRUTH: Not true (thankfully again, for those of us who are reliant on our daily cup of joe). However, caffeine can promote benign breast lumps, cysts, and pain. And I do tell my patients who complain of breast pain or discomfort to try discontinuing caffeine intake (coffee, tea, diet sodas, chocolate), as this may provide some relief from these symptoms.

MYTH: "Cellphone or microwave use can cause breast cancer."

TRUTH: Not true.

MYTH: "Taking birth control pills can cause breast cancer."

TRUTH: Taking birth control pills does not increase the risk of breast cancer. However, it can *decrease* the risk of ovarian cancer.

MYTH: "If you eat all the right things, stay thin, and exercise, there is no chance you can get breast cancer."

TRUTH: The reality is all women are at risk for developing breast cancer regardless of their lifestyle choices.

MYTH: "There is nothing that you can do to decrease your risk of developing breast cancer or decreasing your risk of recurrence if you already have it."

TRUTH: Not precisely true. In fact, being overweight and drinking alcohol regularly can increase the risk of breast cancer and its recurrence. Therefore, maintaining a healthy weight and drinking alcohol in moderation can reduce risk.

MYTH: "If you have a mastectomy, you have a better chance of survival than if you have a lumpectomy with radiation."

TRUTH: For women who are eligible for both operations, lumpectomy and mastectomy are associated with equivalent survival rates.

MYTH: "You can't get breast cancer again after a mastectomy."

TRUTH: The risk of systemic breast cancer recurrence (when the cancer comes back in another part of the body) is the same for women who have mastectomy as have lumpectomy. In addition, breast cancer can recur in the remaining skin or residual breast tissue even after a mastectomy.

MYTH: "Men can't get breast cancer."

TRUTH: Approximately 2,500 men are diagnosed with breast cancer each year in the United States. They account for less than 1 percent of all new breast cancer diagnoses, and less than 1 percent of all new cancer cases in men.

MYTH: "If cancer has spread to the lymph nodes, then mastectomy is a better choice than lumpectomy."

TRUTH: Positively not true, and many patients are surprised to hear this. Having positive lymph nodes may mean that more lymph nodes need to be removed, but it does *not* mean that more tissue needs to be taken from the breast. As long as lumpectomy with clear margins can be achieved in the same way that we would desire for a woman with negative nodes, lumpectomy is perfectly acceptable for women with positive nodes as well.

Appendix 2

frequently asked questions: friends and family

When you are a close family member or friend of someone diagnosed with breast cancer, you're likely to have many questions. What's your role? How can you help? When should you be available and when do you need to take a step back? There is no question that the emotional aspect of caring for someone undergoing breast cancer treatment can be complex. For most of my patients' families and friends, however, it's the implications of the disease and the practicalities of their role as caregiver that concern them the most. Here are some frequently asked questions that I hear from family and friends of my patients, and some of my answers.

1. Does my mother's/sister's/daughter's diagnosis affect me and my risk of getting breast cancer?

The answer is yes, now that you have a family history of breast cancer, your risk is increased. This increased risk can be marginal or significant—it depends on a number of different factors. How old was your relative when she was diagnosed? Did she have other risk factors that affected *only* her? Does your family have a genetic predisposition? It's a good idea to seek counsel from your own doctor regarding your specific level of risk and what this will mean in terms of your screening schedule. It's not always appropriate—and sometimes awkward—to ask your relative's doctor to answer questions about *your* risk when you are not the patient. (For more on determining your own risk, go to chapter 1.)

2. When my friend/relative is receiving chemotherapy, is it safe for me to be around her? Is it safe for her to be around me? What about having small children in the room?

Yes, it is safe to be around your friend or relative when she's having chemotherapy. Thankfully, there is no way of "catching" breast cancer treatment! However, patients receiving chemotherapy *are* at increased risk of infection, as their immune systems are somewhat compromised, and as a result, they should avoid being around others who are sick or have any communicable illnesses. It's important to be honest and up front with your friend or family member if you are not feeling well. Don't visit because you feel you have to—in fact, the best thing you can do for your friend or relative is to stay at home when you're sick. If possible, patients receiving chemotherapy should be shielded from children who are sick or who bring home bugs from school, but of course this isn't always feasible for mothers undergoing treatment. (For more on chemotherapy, go to chapter 9.)

3. Are patients who are receiving radiation for breast cancer radioactive? Can the treatment be damaging or affect others around them?

There are some types of radiation treatment—for example, when people receive treatment for thyroid cancer—where the radiation can be transmitted to others, and where patients are typically quarantined in the hospital to avoid exposure to others. This is not the case for breast cancer. It is completely safe for people of all ages to be around patients receiving radiation for breast cancer, and there is no risk of radiation being transmitted to others. (For more on radiation, go to chapter 10.)

4. Does someone need to stay with my friend/family member when she comes home from the hospital after surgery?

Recovery from breast cancer surgery is quite variable and depends on the specific operation being done. I usually recommend that for the first night or two after the patient goes home, they should not stay alone in case of emergency. Complications from breast cancer surgery are very rare, but the patient will have some restricted mobility in the upper body, and heaven forbid something unexpected should happen around the house while they are still unable to move fully. Equally, for the patient, having someone around for the first couple of days can be a great source of support. For more on the recovery period, go to chapter 12; also see my answer to question 6 below.

5. My wife/sister/mother is having breast cancer surgery, and the sight of blood (or any body fluid) makes me queasy. Will she need the kind of help that will involve seeing the wounds or blood, and if so, what should I do? I don't want to let her down!

Many people are uncomfortable with the sight of blood. I knew two fellow students in medical school who made it through the entire first year before figuring out that being in the operating room and around blood made them faint. (One dropped out of medical school and the other got over it and went on to become a well-known surgeon!) The key is to be aware of your comfort level in advance and to plan accordingly. Some women (and almost all who have mastectomies) leave the hospital after surgery with drains in place. These need to be emptied of bloody fluid, and the output needs to recorded. If the thought of performing this task makes you uneasy, don't do it; enlist someone else. You will do more harm than good when your wife or mother or sister has to call 911 because you fainted, collapsed, and hit your head. If no one else is available to help, there are often visiting nurse services that are available who can come to the house once or twice a day to perform this task; your surgeon's office may be able to help arrange this.

6. How long does recovery from surgery take?

Recovering from breast surgery depends to a large degree on the type of surgery the woman receives. Lumpectomy or mastectomy? Mastectomy on one side or both sides? Sentinel node biopsy or axillary dissection?

For patients who are having a lumpectomy alone, or a lumpectomy and sentinel node biopsy, the recovery process is fairly short. Patients come into the hospital on the morning of surgery, surgery usually takes approximately one hour, and they can go home that evening. Most women do not require significant amounts of pain medication or care. They may have some limited range of motion and soreness in the operated arm if a sentinel node biopsy was performed, but this usually doesn't last long. I have patients with desk jobs who have this type of surgery on Thursday and are back to work on Monday. If the patient's job involves heavy lifting or physical labor, however, it could be three to four weeks before she is able to resume her full duties.

For women who have mastectomies or bilateral mastectomies, recovery can take much longer than with lumpectomy, and usually includes at least an overnight hospital stay. In these cases, it's usually at least two to three weeks before the patient can go back to work, perhaps longer when work involves physical activity. The type of reconstruction received after mastectomy is also a major factor in the recovery length. With implants, a woman can be up and out of bed even on the day of surgery and able to eat and drink (if she's not nauseated from anesthesia). With flap reconstruction, however, recovery is significantly longer, as this surgery involves taking skin and tissue from another site, usually the belly, and as a result, it involves recovering from chest *and* abdominal surgery at the same time. Patients are usually fairly immobile for a day or more, and the road to full recovery can be a longer one, anywhere from six to eight weeks.

Underlying health factors play a big role in recovery duration too. Younger, healthier patients tend to bounce back more quickly and are usually much more resilient, but I certainly see many spry older patients who recover quickly as well. Throughout the healing process, it's important to encourage your loved one to pace herself, and take as much time as she needs to recover. (For more on recovery time frames, go to chapters 6 and 12.)

7. How long after surgery does additional treatment (chemotherapy or radiation) usually start?

Before either chemotherapy or radiation can begin, patients need at least a few weeks to recover and to allow wounds from surgery to heal. If the patient needs chemotherapy, then this is usually the first treatment to follow surgery, before radiation (chemo and radiation are not given concurrently). After chemo is completed, then radiation can begin a few weeks after that. For patients who aren't having chemotherapy, they can move on and start radiation directly, a few weeks after surgery. Anti-hormonal therapy also does not begin until both chemotherapy and radiation are completed, and is thus usually the last form of treatment in the overall course.

For women who are having neoadjuvant chemotherapy (chemotherapy before surgery; see chapter 9 for more on this) the same is true—it's just that the order of treatments is changed. We typically don't do any surgery until a few weeks after chemotherapy is completed, and subsequent treatments follow after that. For more on chemotherapy treatment schedules, go to chapter 9.

8. Will my family member/friend/loved one feel sick during chemotherapy? Will she be able to work? Will she lose her hair?

Different chemotherapy regimens affect different women in different ways. Some patients cruise through chemotherapy with only a few bad days; others find they have to spend a substantial amount of time resting and recovering after each session of treatment. Keep in mind that chemotherapy is given in cycles every one, two, or three weeks, and patients may feel their worst two to three days after the treatment.

Many patients do continue to work during chemotherapy and find work to be a welcome diversion, helping them to maintain a sense of normalcy. Others may want to take the opportunity to rest and focus on recovery during this time. Much depends on the nature of the work, and if it's possible to take a substantial amount of time away from it. Patients who are receiving chemotherapy are at increased risk for infection, so serious and extensive exposures should be avoided if at all possible—I have many patients who are teachers and during the winter months, putting a chemotherapy patient inside a classroom of children with runny noses might not be the best idea. Any work that involves a large amount of physical activity may also be challenging. I have had patients who are waitresses who really needed to cut back on their shifts, finding that all the hours on their feet, clearing plates and lifting trays, was just too much for them. Many people have the option of working from home or telecommuting, which can be helpful during chemotherapy when it's hard to predict how you will feel from day to day. For more on chemotherapy treatment, go to chapter 9.

Hair loss, associated with most but not all types of chemotherapy, while not a significant medical side effect, often has the strongest emotional and psychological impact on a patient. Reminding your loved one that hair loss is a temporary state, and encouraging her to go out and carry on as best as possible with a wig, a scarf, a hat, or nothing at all, is the best support you can give.

Online Resources

G oing online is a part of the information-seeking process for many
women newly diagnosed with breast cancer, and you or your family
members may search out information at various points in your course of
treatment. Should you choose to refer to online resources there are many
that are reputable and up to date, but I hope that the information in this
book has driven home the point that online information acquisition is usually limited by the inability to discern what, if anything, you are reading is
relevant to your particular case. The sources listed below are trusted, but
again, even reputable sources cannot usually provide individually tailored
information or advice. Here is a list of some useful online resources, which
are all the more helpful when you have a top-notch team advising you
about how the information you might find relates to your particular case:

PubMed
http://www.ncbi.nlm.nih.gov/pubmed
Want to know what doctors are reading? This resource, providing
access to scientific publications in peer-reviewed journals, forms the
basis of most of medical literature. While it may be tough to decipher our language without a medical background, most people can
understand the basics. You can search by topic or by author if you

are interested in reading about an individual doctor's particular research interests or accomplishments.

American Cancer Society
http://www.cancer.org
Both information and important resources for people with all types of cancer.

National Cancer Institute (NCI) of the National Institutes of Health (NIH)
http://www.cancer.gov
Reliable information about all kinds of cancer, including breast, with a focus on research.

NCI Clinical Trials Registry
http://www.cancer.gov/clinicaltrials/search
An excellent way to search for clinical trials for breast cancer at the NCI, in all parts of the country, or in your geographic area specifically.

NCI SEER (Surveillance, Epidemiology, End Results) Program
http://seer.cancer.gov/statfacts/html/breast.html
Provides current facts on breast cancer, including numbers of cases and survival data.

The Oncofertility Consortium
http://oncofertility.northwestern.edu
Many resources for women of childbearing age interested in fertility preservation.

Save My Fertility
http://www.savemyfertility.org
A resource for women of childbearing age, providing information on fertility preservation.

The American Society of Clinical Oncology
http://www.asco.org
The leading national association of medical oncologists. Has a useful online directory for identifying practitioners in your area or from any part of the world. Also an excellent resource for practice quality

guidelines, mostly for physicians, but certainly accessible to the lay public as well.

The Susan G. Komen Foundation

http://ww5.komen.org

A nationally recognized resource for information about breast cancer, research, and support efforts.

The Breast Cancer Research Foundation

http://www.bcrfcure.org

Founded by Evelyn Lauder, one of the leading philanthropic sources of breast cancer research funding for the field's leaders and their efforts. Also has an excellent facts and resources section at http://www.bcrfcure.org/breast-cancer-statistics-resources.

The Gail Model Risk Assessment Tool

http://www.cancer.gov/bcrisktool/

This model is used by many physicians to assess risk for breast cancer, and can help guide decisions regarding the need for added screening and prevention strategies.

FDA

http://www.accessdata.fda.gov/scripts/cdrh/cfdocs/cfMQSA/mqsa.cfm

This website provides information by geographic area on FDA approved mammogram facilities across the country.

The Society for Integrative Oncology

http://www.integrativeonc.org

If you are interested in finding out more or incorporating integrative medicine approaches into your care, this website is a resource for evidence-based information.

Glossary of Terms

Three-dimensional (3-D) mammography Newer mammographic technique that sections through the breast rather than taking single pictures. Reduces call-back rates for potential abnormalities by eliminating false positives related to tissue overlap. Slightly higher radiation exposure per examination.

Adenoid cystic carcinoma Rare subtype of breast cancer.

Alcohol intake The amount of alcohol you consume, typically measured as drinks per day (one shot of alcohol, one glass of wine, and one beer each equal one drink). More than one to two drinks per day (more than seven to ten per week) is thought to increase your risk of developing breast cancer and, for women with breast cancer, increase risk of recurrence. Recommendations are for moderate alcohol intake at most: no more than five drinks per week.

Alternative medicine Treatments or therapies that are outside of standard proven medical modalities for treating disease, often chosen in lieu of standard treatment.

Anti-hormonal therapy Synonymous with "Endocrine therapy." Medical treatment, usually in pill form, that treats estrogen-receptor-positive (ER-positive) breast cancer. Used to treat in a variety of different settings: (1) for metastatic breast cancer to control disease,

(2) to reduce the risk of breast cancer recurrence for cancers that are ER-positive, and (3) to prevent breast cancer in women at increased risk for developing the disease. See also "Aromatase inhibitors" and "Tamoxifen."

Areola The darker-colored skin circle on the breast surrounding the nipple.

Aromatase inhibitors (AI) A class of anti-hormonal therapy drugs that work by reducing estrogen production by the body. Only effective in postmenopausal women. See also "Endocrine therapy," "Anti-hormonal therapy," and "Tamoxifen."

Asymmetry An area of distortion seen on the mammogram that is not symmetric with the surrounding breast tissue or with the other side. Asymmetry suggests something is pulling or distorting the surrounding tissue. Can be caused by many things, such as a scar from a previous biopsy or injury, but also can be a sign of cancer. Usually requires further evaluation, especially if new when compared to previous images. See also "Density," "Mass," and "Lump."

Atypia or atypical hyperplasia (includes atypical ductal hyperplasia and atypical lobular hyperplasia) A specific type of change to cells that can be seen under the microscope when breast tissue is examined, showing cells that are "atypical," or not typical-looking. Can be seen adjacent to areas of cancer; thus atypia seen on a needle biopsy usually warrants a small surgery or excision of the surrounding area to make sure there is no cancer present. The finding of atypia does mean a moderately increased risk of future breast cancer, approximately 15 percent over one's lifetime. See also "Tamoxifen."

Autologous tissue The use of one's own tissue to reconstruct a breast removed by mastectomy. Most common site from which tissue is taken is from the belly, but other sites can include the buttocks and the back. See also "DIEP flap" and "Latissimus dorsi flap."

Axillary lymph node(s) Lymph nodes in the armpit that drain the arm and breast on that side. These are checked in the setting of invasive breast cancer and sometimes with DCIS to find out if cancer has spread.

Axillary lymph node dissection Operation performed to remove all the lymph nodes in the armpit. Done in some cases when cancer has been found to have spread there.

Baseline mammogram First-ever mammogram. Usually recommended at age forty, sometimes earlier if there is a family history of breast cancer diagnosed at a young age.

Benign Not cancer; normal finding on biopsy.

Bilateral Both sides, usually referring to both left and right breast. See also "Bilateral mastectomy" and "Double mastectomy."

Bilateral mastectomy Synonymous with "Double mastectomy." Removal of both breasts, can be done in the setting of prevention of breast cancer, when one breast has cancer and the other, normal breast is also electively removed, or in the rare setting of breast cancer diagnosed on both sides.

Biopsy Removal of a piece of tissue to look at it under the microscope, test it, and make a diagnosis. Can be a small piece (see also "Needle biopsy") or a larger piece (see also "Surgical biopsy" and "Excision").

Bone scan A test done to determine if breast cancer has spread or metastasized to bones.

BRCA-1 A gene that when mutated or abnormal is associated with an increased risk of developing breast cancer (approximately 80 percent), ovarian cancer (20 to 40 percent), and other cancers to a lesser degree. BRCA-1 cancers are frequently triple negative. See also "Genetic testing," "Genetic counseling," and "Triple negative."

BRCA-2 A gene that when mutated or abnormal is associated with an increased risk of developing breast cancer (approximately 80 percent), ovarian cancer (10 to 20 percent), and other cancers to a lesser degree. Compared to BRCA-1, BRCA-2 cancers are more frequently ER-positive. See also "Genetic testing" and "Genetic counseling."

Breast cancer The result when breast cell changes at the genetic level lead a cell to grow, divide, multiply, and spread without normal controls. See also "Tumor."

Calcifications Deposits of calcium seen as clusters of tiny white spots on a mammogram. Can be the first sign of breast cancer (20 percent), but also can be related to normal findings (80 percent).

CAT or CT scan A scan that can be done of a particular part or region of the body to look for breast cancer spread. Often done of the chest, abdomen, and pelvis to look for breast cancer spread in the lungs and liver. Often done in combination with a bone scan. See also "PET scan" and "Bone scan."

Chemo-brain Cognitive or neurologic changes, such as difficulties with memory, recall, or thinking process, attributed to chemotherapy.

Chemotherapy/systemic therapy Medicine, specifically chemical substances, aimed at killing cancer cells given to treat breast cancer or reduce its risk of recurrence. Usually given intravenously, occasionally orally.

Clinical trial A scientific, controlled test to determine the effectiveness of a new option for treatment before it can be made available to the general public and offered as a standard option for treatment.

Complementary medicine Treatments or therapies that are outside of standard proven medical modalities for treating disease, are often combined with standard treatments, and are aimed at alleviating symptoms related to standard treatments or disease.

Contralateral (prophylactic or risk-reducing) mastectomy Removal of the other, normal breast in addition to the one with cancer. Usually done with the intent of reducing the risk of getting breast cancer on the other side. Also done in some cases to eliminate the need for future imaging and possibly biopsy, and sometimes with the goal of achieving a more symmetrical cosmetic result. See also "Risk-reducing mastectomy."

Core needle biopsy Procedure of choice to take small snippets of tissue of a suspicious area in order to make a diagnosis. Involves local anesthesia and taking small cores or pieces of tissue from a suspicious area. See also "Stereotactic biopsy," "Mammotome biopsy," "MRI-guided core biopsy," and "Ultrasound-guided core biopsy."

Cyst (simple cyst) A fluid-filled pocket in the breast that is a completely normal finding. One potential cause of a new mass that one feels in the breast.

DCIS (Ductal Carcinoma-in-situ) Noninvasive breast cancer, also referred to as stage 0 breast cancer.

Dense tissue Breast tissue that is thick and firm, and appears whiter on mammogram than its counterpart, fatty tissue. A new cancer can be obscured and difficult to identify against a background of dense tissue.

Density A descriptive word used to describe a mass or whiter area seen on a mammogram or other study, usually indicating the need for further follow-up studies. A density can prove to be normal or cancer. See also "Asymmetry," "Mass," and "Lump."

Diagnostic test Any type of radiology test to further evaluate abnormal findings on either physical examination or prior imaging test. See also "Screening test."

DIEP flap Type of reconstruction using one's own tissue from the lower abdomen to rebuild the breast. The deep inferior epigastric perforator (DIEP) vessels of the abdomen are connected to vessels in the chest for blood supply.

Double mastectomy Synonymous with "Bilateral mastectomy." Removing both breasts. Usually performed for cancer on one side with removal of the other, normal breast by choice. Can also be performed to reduce risk of developing breast cancer in high-risk situations, or in the rare situation of breast cancer diagnosed on both sides. See also "Unilateral mastectomy" and "Risk-reducing mastectomy."

Duct lavage A test that involves injecting fluid into the nipple and duct system of the breast and aspirating the fluid along with cells lining the duct. The test was purported to determine the risk of developing breast cancer and even possibly diagnosing breast cancer. In practice, the test was never appropriately validated, and the significance of the results could not be definitively determined. As a result, duct lavage fell out of favor and is no longer routinely used or recommended.

Endocrine therapy Synonymous with "Anti-hormonal therapy." Medical treatment, usually in pill form, that treats estrogen-receptor-positive breast cancer. Used in a variety of different settings: (1) for metastatic breast cancer to control disease, (2) to reduce the risk of breast cancer recurrence for cancers that are estrogen-receptor-positive, and (3) to prevent breast cancer in women at increased risk for developing the disease. See also "Aromatase inhibitors" and "Tamoxifen."

Estrogen/progesterone-receptor-negative Terminology used to describe a tumor that does not have estrogen or progesterone receptors on the cells' surfaces, and therefore does not respond to and cannot be treated with anti-hormonal or endocrine therapy. See also "Aromatase inhibitors," "Tamoxifen," "Endocrine therapy," and "Anti-hormonal therapy."

Estrogen/progesterone-receptor-positive Terminology used to describe a tumor that has a measurable number of estrogen or progesterone receptors on its cells' surfaces, and therefore responds to and can be treated with anti-hormonal or endocrine therapy.

Excision Removal of tissue for the purpose of establishing a diagnosis or to completely remove a designated area via a surgical procedure.

Family history Having relatives who have had breast cancer. See also "First-degree relative" and "Second-degree relative."

Fellowship Advanced training to specialize in a particular area of expertise. For example, breast surgery fellowship involves one to two years of additional training in breast surgery beyond the standard five-year general surgery training period.

Fibroadenoma One of the most common causes of a benign breast lump, especially in young women. Not associated with cancer or an increased risk of cancer.

Fibrocystic disease/fibrocystic changes A condition of benign breast tissue that can cause normal lumps, bumps, and cysts. Very common among premenopausal women.

Fine needle aspiration (FNA) A type of needle biopsy that aspirates cells from an area to get a preliminary determination of whether or not an area is abnormal. Limited by the small amount of cells that can be removed. Differs from a core biopsy, which can remove actual pieces of tissue and can give a definitive result. See also "Core needle biopsy."

First-degree relative Parent, sibling, or child. See also "Second-degree relative."

Gail model A mathematical model used to calculate approximate risk of an individual for developing breast cancer.

General anesthesia Anesthesia that affects the whole body and involves loss of consciousness. Can include intubation (placement of a breathing tube). See also "Local anesthesia."

Genetic counseling Meeting with a trained, certified genetic counselor who evaluates one's family history of cancer, the ages at which cancer developed, and the types of cancer to determine the likelihood of having an identifiable hereditary syndrome predisposing to cancer. Will also counsel regarding the risks and benefits of genetic testing.

Genetic testing Blood or saliva test (to obtain DNA) to determine the presence of a genetic mutation that predisposes one to an increased risk of a specific cancer or cancers.

Her2/neu A tumor gene that is amplified or overexpressed in approximately 15 to 20 percent of breast cancers. Herceptin and other medications specifically target these tumors and reduce their risk of recurrence in combination with chemotherapy. Her2/neu-positive tumors are often considered when giving chemotherapy before surgery. See also "Neoadjuvant chemotherapy" and "Herceptin."

Herceptin Medicine given that specifically targets Her2/neu-positive tumors.

Hormone receptors Found on the cell surface of cancers that are hormone-receptor positive. Cancers with hormone receptors need circulating hormones to grow and spread. Medications such as tamoxifen function to block hormone receptors and prevent growth. See also "Tamoxifen" and "Aromatase inhibitors."

Hospice care End-of-life care when death is imminent. Usually involves pain control, support for basic functions, and psychological, emotional, and spiritual support for patients and their families. See also "Palliative care."

Implant Silicone- or saline-filled capsule that is used to reconstruct the breast after mastectomy.

Indeterminate Results from a needle biopsy that are inconclusive and usually require removal of the area with surgery to obtain a definitive diagnosis.

Inflammatory breast cancer An aggressive form of breast cancer characterized by involvement of the breast and overlying skin. Treatment involves chemotherapy first, followed by surgery, and radiation.

Invasive/infiltrating ductal cancer The most common type of invasive breast cancer, accounting for approximately 80 percent of all cases. See also "Invasive/infiltrating lobular cancer" and "DCIS."

Invasive/infiltrating lobular cancer The second most common type of invasive breast cancer, accounting for approximately 10 percent of all cases. Invasive lobular cancers can be more difficult to detect mammographically, and can thus be associated with larger tumor size.

Latissimus dorsi flap Type of reconstruction using one's own tissue from the latissimus dorsi muscle in the back, overlying the shoulder blade. See also "Autologous tissue" and "DIEP flap."

LCIS or lobular carcinoma in situ Cell changes that are not cancer but indicate a higher risk of developing a future breast cancer over one's lifetime, approximately 20 percent.

Li-Fraumeni syndrome Rare genetic syndrome that predisposes to breast cancer, sarcoma, brain tumors, leukemia, and others.

Local anesthesia Anesthesia that affects only one isolated part of the body. Frequently used for breast biopsies and smaller breast procedures.

Local recurrence Breast cancer that comes back in the affected breast after previous lumpectomy.

Localization procedure Placement of a needle or seed in the breast prior to surgery to lead the surgeon to an area targeted for removal.

Lump A prominent area that can be felt on physical exam that stands out against the rest of the breast. See also "Mass."

Lumpectomy One option for breast cancer surgery that removes a small part of the breast. Often coupled with radiation treatment to follow.

Lymph node Glands that are filled with immune system cells and to which cancer can spread. Can be found in groups and basins throughout the body, including in the neck, armpits, and groin.

Lymphatics Tiny threadlike vessels through which lymph fluid flows toward lymph nodes. One of the main pathways for cancer spread.

Lymphedema Swelling of the arm that can develop when axillary (armpit) lymph nodes are removed from that side.

Lynch syndrome A rare genetic mutation that predisposes to colon, uterine, and breast cancer.

Magnification views Additional specialized mammogram pictures that magnify an area of concern, done especially when concerned about or to get a better view of calcifications.

Malignant/malignancy Pertaining to cancer.

Mammogram A radiologic study done for breast cancer detection. The only test that has been shown to reduce the risk of mortality from breast cancer.

Mammotome biopsy A needle biopsy technique guided by findings seen on a mammogram.

Mantle radiation A type of radiation treatment given to the chest wall for Hodgkin's disease (lymphoma). When given, especially in the teenage years, can significantly increase risk of developing a future breast cancer, and warrants high-risk screening.

Margin The rim of tissue around a tumor that is removed. A negative margin indicates there is normal tissue surrounding the cancer suggesting that the tumor was completely removed. A positive margin indicates that cancer cells came up to the edge of the tissue removed, thereby raising concern that there is residual cancer still left in the breast. Usually applies to lumpectomy surgery. See also "Re-excision."

Mass A lump or bump in the breast tissue that can be either felt or seen on imaging studies. See also "Lump."

Mastectomy One option for breast cancer surgery that removes all of the breast tissue and usually the nipple. Also can be done to prevent breast cancer in those at high risk.

Medullary cancer A subtype of breast cancer.

Metastasis/metastatic disease Spread of breast cancer outside the breast. Distant metastatic disease is spread to other parts of the body, most commonly lungs, liver, bone, and brain.

Microcalcifications Tiny white spots seen on a mammogram that are calcium deposits. May be a sign of breast cancer. If new or changed, usually require a biopsy. See also "Mammogram," "Stereotactic biopsy," and "Mammotome biopsy."

Modified radical mastectomy Removal of all breast tissue, nipple, and areola, coupled with removal of axillary nodes. Done in cases where mastectomy is being performed and there is also spread to axillary lymph nodes thereby indicating the need for removal. Can be synonymous with "Skin-sparing mastectomy" when most of the skin envelope is also preserved. See also "Simple mastectomy."

Mortality Death or risk of dying.

MRI A radiology examination used in screening for breast cancer in high-risk populations. Also used in determining extent of disease in the breast for selected women already diagnosed with breast cancer.

MRI-guided core biopsy A needle biopsy performed with MRI guidance to sample an abnormality seen on MRI.

Mucinous cancer Subtype of breast cancer, usually associated with good prognosis.

Neoadjuvant chemotherapy Chemotherapy that is given before surgery to shrink a breast cancer. Usually given with the goal of making subsequent surgery more likely to be successful in advanced cases, or with the goal of increasing the chance of successful lumpectomy for a larger tumor. Also commonly given in cases of triple negative or Her2/neu-positive breast cancer. See also "Triple negative" and "Her2/neu."

Neuropathy Potential side effect of some chemotherapy drugs that involves pain, numbness, or weakness in the limbs or extremities.

Nipple inversion Nipple that is pulled inward instead of projecting outward. Can be normal and long-standing, or can be a symptom of breast cancer, particularly when new or changed, due to a tumor behind the nipple pulling it in.

Nipple-sparing mastectomy A variation of mastectomy that involves sparing the nipple and surrounding areola. Eliminates the need for nipple reconstruction.

Nodule Descriptive word usually used to describe a small mass or lump that is more likely to be benign.

Obesity Extreme of being overweight. Associated with increased risk of breast cancer and an increased risk of breast cancer recurrence for those already diagnosed.

Occult breast cancer Approximately 1 percent of all breast cancer cases, where the first sign of breast cancer is a cancerous node under the arm, with no identifiable source of cancer in the breast based on examination or mammogram.

Oncofertility Subspecialty of fertility medicine focused on reproductive options and fertility preservation and safety in cancer survivors.

Oncologist: medical, surgical, radiation Physician who specializes in the care and treatment of patients with cancer using medicine, surgery, or radiation, depending on specialty.

Oncotype DX A genetic profile of a tumor stratifying it at high, intermediate, or low risk of recurrence. Used in selected patients to help determine need for chemotherapy.

Overdiagnosis Diagnosing a disease or condition that would never become a health issue if left alone.

Paget's disease A subtype of breast cancer that involves the nipple.

Palliative care An approach that focuses on pain and symptom control for patients with severe and life-threatening disease.

Pathologist/pathology Specialist or specialty that examines tissue to determine diagnosis.

Peau d'orange Literally "skin of an orange." Breast skin changes including thickening and pitting that are signs of inflammatory breast cancer.

Perjeta A new drug targeting Her2/neu-positive breast cancer, frequently given in combination with Herceptin. See also "Her2/neu" and "Herceptin."

PET scan/PET-CT A total body scan (frequently coupled with CT scan) that is performed to look for metastatic disease or spread of cancer in the body. Can also be used in patients with known metastatic disease to assess response to treatment.

Placebo A substance, pill, or treatment that has no therapeutic effect. Frequently used in one arm of a trial to compare effects and side effects of an actual treatment in the other arm.

Post-mastectomy radiation Radiation given after mastectomy, usually in cases of large or locally advanced tumors or extensive lymph node involvement.

Prognosis The likely or expected course or outcome of a disease.

Prophylactic mastectomy Removal of a breast to prevent breast cancer. See also "Risk-reducing mastectomy."

Prosthesis A breast-shaped piece of material, usually made of silicone or fabric, that can be placed in the bra to fill it out after a mastectomy in lieu of reconstruction.

Radiation/radiation oncologist A treatment for breast cancer and the physician who plans and administers the treatment, usually after lumpectomy, occasionally after mastectomy.

Radical mastectomy An operation performed for breast cancer, rarely done and needed in the current era, which involves removing the breast, lymph nodes, and the underlying pectoralis muscle.

Radiologist A physician who reads and interprets imaging studies such as mammograms, ultrasounds, MRIs, X-rays, and CAT scans.

Randomization The process of assigning people or patients to different groups of a study without bias so that study groups will be even in terms of patient population and characteristics.

Reconstruction The process of rebuilding and re-forming the breast after mastectomy. See also "DIEP flap," "Implant," and "Latissimus dorsi flap."

Recurrence When breast cancer returns after treatment and a disease-free interval. See also "Local recurrence" and "Systemic recurrence."

Re-excision The procedure of removing additional tissue after lumpectomy when margins are not clear of cancer. See also "Margin."

Risk-reducing mastectomy Removing the breast or breasts when no cancer is present to reduce the risk of developing a future cancer in that breast. See also "Contralateral mastectomy" and "Prophylactic mastectomy."

Screening test A test done in people with no symptoms with the goal of detecting a disease. See also "Mammogram" and "Diagnostic test."

Second-degree relative Grandparent, aunt/uncle, grandchild, niece/nephew.

Self-examination Examining oneself for signs of an illness. With breast self-examination, focuses especially on lumps, skin, or nipple changes.

Sentinel lymph node (biopsy) Standard procedure for examining lymph nodes under the arm for spread of cancer. See also "Axillary lymph node dissection."

Side effect Consequence of a treatment or intervention that is usually undesirable.

Simple mastectomy Removal of all breast tissue, nipple, and areola. Can be synonymous with "Skin-sparing mastectomy" when most of the skin envelope is also preserved. Synonymous with "Total mastectomy." See also "Skin-sparing mastectomy" and "Modified radical mastectomy."

Simulation The planning phase of radiation.

Skin dimpling Visible indentation of the skin, raising the concern for the presence of a cancer underneath pulling the skin inward.

Skin-sparing mastectomy Removal of all the breast tissue, nipple, and areola while preserving most of the surrounding skin envelope for improved cosmetic result. See also "Simple mastectomy" and "Modified radical mastectomy."

Sonogram (synonymous with "Ultrasound") A medical imaging test using high-frequency sound waves to delineate structures in the body. Particularly useful for differentiating fluid (as in a cyst) from solid (as with a mass).

Specialization Additional training to develop expertise in a particular field. See also "Fellowship."

Stage/staging A system that is used to estimate cancer prognosis. For breast cancer, TNM staging is used, which involves tumor size, lymph node status, and presence or absence of distant metastatic disease.

Stage 0 DCIS (noninvasive cancer) only.

Stage 1 Invasive cancer with tumor size 2 centimeters or less and no lymph node involvement.

Stage 2 Invasive cancer with tumor size greater than 2 centimeters and/or lymph node involvement.

Stage 3 Larger tumor size, more extensive lymph node involvement, or tumor that is more locally advanced, including overlying skin involvement or underlying pectoralis muscle invasion. Also includes inflammatory breast cancer (categorized as stage 3B) and breast cancer involving lymph nodes above the collar bone (categorized as stage 3C).

Stage 4 Breast cancer that has spread (metastasized) to distant sites in the body, most commonly lung, liver, bone, and brain.

Stereotactic biopsy Needle biopsy guided by findings on a mammogram. Synonymous with "Mammotome biopsy."

Surgical biopsy Removal of tissue to establish a diagnosis via a surgical procedure.

Survivorship Transition period after treatment when there is no evidence of recurrence and focus shifts toward maintenance of overall general and continued surveillance for recurrence.

Systemic recurrence Breast cancer return to the body. Synonymous with Stage 4.

Tamoxifen Medication given for hormone-receptor-positive disease to reduce the risk of recurrence.

Thermography An experimental test with the goal of differentiating malignancy from normal findings by analyzing heat distribution.

Tissue expander Temporary device inserted at the time of mastectomy as part of the initial stage of the reconstruction process.

Total mastectomy Removal of all breast tissue, nipple and areola. Can be synonymous with "Skin-sparing mastectomy" when most of the skin envelope is also preserved. Synonymous with "Simple mastectomy." See also "Skin-sparing mastectomy" and "Modified radical mastectomy."

Triple negative Breast cancer that does not express estrogen, progesterone, or Her2/neu receptor.

Tubular cancer Subtype of breast cancer typically associated with lower likelihood of spread and better prognosis.

Tumor An abnormal growth of tissue, usually associated with malignancy, but can also be benign.

Tumor grade Description of cancer cells that indicates how abnormal the cells look compared to normal cells. Often, but not always, an indicator of cell growth, spread, and aggressiveness.

Tumor marker A substance found in the blood or urine that can be an indicator of the presence of cancer or recurrence.

Ultrasound A medical imaging test using high-frequency sound waves to delineate structures in the body. Particularly useful for differentiating fluid (as in a cyst) from solid (as with a mass). Synonymous with "Sonogram."

Ultrasound-guided core biopsy Needle biopsy guided by an ultrasound or sonogram finding.

Underdiagnosis Failure of a test to detect a disease that is clinically significant and will affect overall health. See also "Overdiagnosis."

Unilateral One side or one breast. See also "Bilateral" and "Contralateral mastectomy."

Unilateral mastectomy Removal of one breast. See also "bilateral" and "bilateral mastectomy."

Z-11 trial Landmark trial in breast cancer showing that for most women who have had a lumpectomy and have one or two positive nodes, removing the rest of the nodes (axillary dissection) is not necessary due to the low risk of residual disease, and the likelihood that additional treatments including chemotherapy, anti-hormonal therapy, and radiation will eradicate any residual disease.

Index

Herceptin, 126, 137, 279, 282
high-volume centers, xiv–xv, 58, 61–62, 64–65, 115, 133–34, 243
Hodgkin's disease, 14–15, 160
hormonal sensitivity, 39
hormonal therapy, 15–16, 95, 125, 132, 146–50, 250
  with chemotherapy, 150
  duration, 148
  male breast cancer, 218
  obesity, 186
  recovery period, 175
  recurrence of breast cancer, 237
  side effects, 148–50, 175
hormone exposure, 13
  birth control pills, 261
  pregnancy, 42, 226
hormone receptor status, 124–27, 129, 146–50, 277, 279
  biopsies, 39, 153
  male breast cancer, 218–19
  metastatic breast cancer, 240
  obesity, 185–86
  Oncotype DX assay, 151–52
hormone replacement therapy, 13
hospice, 247, 279
hypnosis, 194

image-guided biopsies, 32–33
immune system, 72, 74
  stress, 189–90
  suppression, 142
  See also lymph nodes
implant reconstruction, 111–12, 114, 158, 172, 279
indeterminate results, 39–40, 279
infiltrating cancer. *See* invasive breast cancer
inflammatory breast cancer, 69, 77, 105–6, 129–30, 279
  mastectomy and radiation, 161
  neoadjuvant chemotherapy, 153
  reconstruction, 110
informed consent, 166
insulin resistance pathway, 185
insurance. *See* health insurance
integrative medicine. *See* complementary medicine
internal mammary lymph nodes, 73, 130
Internet resources, xi–xii, xvii, xviii, 269–71

interval cancer, 25
invasive breast cancer, 39, 68–69, 279
  chemotherapy, 135
  lumpectomy, 87–89
  lymph node evaluation, 73–79
  mastectomy, 89–92
invasive ductal cancer, 68–69, 279
invasive lobular cancer, 68–69, 279

Ki67 level, 119

late-onset menopause, 13
latissimus dorsi flap, 113, 279
LCIS. *See* lobular carcinoma in situ
leukemia, 144, 175
lifestyle factors, 183–91, 250–51
Li-Fraumeni syndrome, 206, 279
limited resection. *See* lumpectomy
lobular breast cancer, 39, 67–69
lobular carcinoma in situ (LCIS), 13, 15, 279
local anesthesia (def.), 280
localization procedure, 82–83, 280
local recurrence, 235–37, 250, 280
low blood count, 142
lump (def.), 280
lumpectomy, 9, 70–71, 81–85, 280
  advantages and disadvantages, 87–89
  age factors, 95
  bilateral breast cancer, 104–5
  BRCA mutation, 208
  cure and survival rates, 71, 89, 91–92, 100–101
  double lumpectomy, 93–94
  early detection, 9
  follow-up care, 250
  hormonal treatment, 95
  localization procedures, 82–83
  lymph node evaluation, 73, 76
  male breast cancer, 216
  mammograms, 89, 90
  margin status, 120–22
  medical contraindications, 93–95
  need for additional surgery, 87–88, 121–24
  obesity, 186
  orientation of cancer specimen, 84
  orientation of incision, 84, 87, 116
  Paget's disease, 106
  during pregnancy, 225–26